LIZ EARLE'S
QUICK GUIDES
Beating PMS

LIZ EARLE'S
QUICK GUIDES
Beating PMS

B🌾XTREE

Advice to the Reader

Before following any dietary advice contained in this book, it is recommended that you consult your doctor if you suffer from any health problems or special condition or are in any doubt.

First published in Great Britain in 1995 by Boxtree Limited, Broadwall House, 21 Broadwall, London SE1 9PL

The right of Liz Earle to be identified as Author of this Work has been asserted by her in accordance with the Copyright, Designs and Patents Act 1988

10 9 8 7 6 5 4 3 2 1

ISBN: 0 7522 1668 6

Text design by Blackjacks
Cover design by Hammond Hammond

Printed and Bound in Great Britain by Cox & Wyman Ltd., Reading, Berkshire

A CIP catalogue entry for this book is available from the British Library

Contents

ACKNOWLEDGEMENTS

I am grateful to Mandy Piggot and Sarah Hamilton Fleming for helping to produce this book. I am also indebted to the talented team at Boxtree, and to Rosemary Sandberg and Claire Bowles Publicity, for their unfailing enthusiasm and support.

Introduction

Premenstrual syndrome is a fact of life for many women. It can seem to be an illness without a cure. Some doctors are unsympathetic and many are unaware of the relief that can be achieved through simple dietary changes. This *Quick Guide* offers new hope to all those who suffer from the monthly blues. It includes much medically proven advice, and information on the most helpful and up-to-date treatments. Many who have tried the therapies I have detailed have found total relief from PMS symptoms, including depression, irritability, personality changes, mood swings and weight-gain. I would urge all women to read this *Quick Guide* and see just how easy it can be to improve your own quality of life and well-being.

Liz Earle

—— 1 ——

Understanding Premenstrual Syndrome

Could This be You?

There are definitely certain changes that take place a few days before every period, although some months it's worse than others. Physically, my breasts become tender and sore — this always happens and it's what reminds me that my period is due. And my jeans become tighter, in fact it's uncomfortable having anything restrictive around my tummy because it feels so bloated.

Also, this is the time when I am likely to empty the fridge — you know, just run to the kitchen and hoover up all the immediately edible food in sight. Yet I'm not normally a binger, it's just at that particular time.

But the worst thing is this kind of hysterical depression which builds up to a peak the night before my period starts. It's as though there's a black cloud over my head but it's accompanied by a shaky sort of nervous panic, so I want to scream with frustration and despair, rather than just cry. I become convinced that I'm ugly and stupid and my entire life is pointless. I become a nastier person, I snap at people out of pure spite, as though I really want to hurt them, and later I want to cry because I feel so sorry.

When my period starts, sometimes I can actually feel the tension draining away with the flow, as though my whole body's breathing a sigh of relief.

This experience is typical of an estimated ten million women in Britain. They suffer from premenstrual syndrome, or PMS; a collection of physical and mental symptoms that begin anything between two and fourteen days before menstruation, and which are relieved soon after the period starts.

The actual symptoms and their severity will vary widely from woman to woman. For any one individual, the effect of PMS may differ from month to month, but the experience of cyclical symptoms of some description is almost universal amongst women – according to a recent review, mild physiological symptoms occur in 95 percent of women of reproductive age, and for one in twenty the effects are so severe that their lives are totally disrupted once a month.

Why is it so common today? In fact, the phenomenon of mood swings and physical discomforts visiting women premenstrually is as old as the hills, but has only recently been given a name and, with it, a growing credibility. Reading about famous women in years gone by, we can almost certainly spot the symptoms of PMS. Queen Victoria is reported to have screamed and hurled objects at a baffled Prince Albert, who understandably looked forward to her pregnancies, when her behaviour became more settled and predictable; Maria Callas and Judy Garland are both known to have suffered from mood swings and binge eating before their periods.

The psychological effects can be devastating in their violence: suicides, attempted suicides, and acts of aggression against others have all been attributed to premenstrual syndrome.

Nicola Owen made legal history when she was the first woman to use PMS as a mitigating plea in the courts. She was discharged from the Old Bailey, where she had faced charges of arson after trying to commit suicide by setting fire to the family home. Eighteen-year-old Anna Reynolds killed her mother with a hammer but was released on appeal on the strength of medical evidence of the severity of her premenstrual symptoms. Both women's PMS have since responded positively to hormone and dietary treatment.

In 1980, a thirty-six-year-old British woman killed her lover by running him down with her car. The following year, a twenty-eight-year-old barmaid from east London fatally stabbed another woman. Both were charged with murder; both, supported by medical evidence, pleaded the effects of premenstrual syndrome as part of their defence. As a result, both had their charges reduced to manslaughter on the grounds of diminished responsibility and were put on probation, subject to their receiving appropriate treatment.

Thirty percent of women who shop-lift are premenstrual. A study carried out on inmates at Holloway women's prison found that 49 percent of the prisoners had committed their crimes within four days of the start of their period. Even those women who are not driven to crime are more likely to be absent from work, attempt suicide, or be in an accident resulting in admission to hospital, during the days preceding their period.

A Brief History of PMS

Premenstrual symptoms (then known collectively as PMT) were first recorded in 1931, when American Dr Robert Frank observed symptoms of nervous tension, water retention and weight-gain in fifteen women. He attributed this to high levels of oestrogen premenstrually, causing irritation to the nervous system. Shortly afterwards, a similarity with B-vitamin deficiency was observed, and treatment with vitamin B greatly improved symptoms, especially uncomfortable breasts and heavy periods.

The first UK study, in 1937, surveyed 169 women who reported fatigue, headaches and mood swings around the time of their periods. In 1953, Dr Katharina Dalton co-authored the first significant work on the subject in the *British Medical Journal*, and the condition was renamed Premenstrual Syndrome. Dr Dalton went on to spend many years investigating the problem in prisons, hospitals, factories, offices and schools. She blamed the symptoms on low levels of progesterone premenstrually, and treated women successfully using supplements of this hormone.

To date, PMS has been the subject of several thousand research papers and, although doctors have a growing number of treatment strategies at their disposal, we are still a long way from understanding exactly why PMS happens. Current scientific thinking is that most sufferers do not have a hormone imbalance but, rather, are unduly sensitive to the normal swings in hormone levels that occur throughout the menstrual cycle. This sensitivity may in turn be linked to nutrition, so it seems possible to alter that sensitivity, and thus the symptoms, through diet.

So, rather than having a single cause, PMS is more likely to result from a combination of factors with some acting as triggers, while others aggravate symptoms already present.

Although the condition is steadily gaining recognition amongst the medical profession, no single medical speciality has yet accepted responsibility for its treatment. Because it is a 'women's problem', sufferers are most often referred to specialists in obstetrics and gynaecology. But, if this is not successful, the next step is often a psychiatrist, who may in turn send the patient back to the gynaecologist for hormonal treatment.

Who Gets PMS?

The only reliable generalisation that can be made is that only women get PMS! This condition has no respect for class, colour, race, education or economic status. What is more, as well as making many women's lives miserable, it indirectly affects their partners, children, parents, flatmates, employees and work-mates ... and occasionally even unfortunate bystanders.

What are the Symptoms?

All of the symptoms in the following lists have been reported in women premenstrually. One will usually notice that the same symptoms tend to recur, although with varying degrees of severity. There may be changes over time – for example, after having children, the monthly symptoms may become more severe. The type and severity of symptoms tend to vary widely.

Psychological
* Altered sex drive
* Anger and aggression
* Anxiety and panic attacks
* Clumsiness
* Crying uncontrollably, often for no apparent reason
* Depression
* Feelings of insecurity
* Hunger and food cravings, especially for sugary foods
* Irritability
* Loss of control
* Low self-worth
* Mood swings
* Phobias
* Suicidal feelings
* Tension

Physical
* Abdominal bloating and discomfort
* Acne

* Asthma
* Backache
* Breast-swelling or tenderness
* Cold sore recurrence, if already infected
* Dizziness
* Fainting
* Fatigue and loss of energy
* Headaches and migraine
* Joint pains
* Lower back pain
* Nausea or vomiting
* Palpitations
* Rashes
* Runny nose
* Sinusitis
* Sore eyes or throat
* Swollen legs or ankles
* Visual disturbances
* Weight-gain

MOOD CHANGES

I get so irritable that the slightest thing makes me want to snap. The kids don't have to say a word; they only have to be in the same room and I scream at them for being under my feet. Then the next minute I burst into tears for absolutely no reason. It affects everyone around me. In fact, when I discovered I was expecting for the second time, my poor husband said, 'Thank goodness for that!' as he knew he could look forward to a few months of peace!

It was the characteristic feeling of tension – like a coiled-up spring ready to explode with anger at the slightest provocation – that lent itself to the name 'premenstrual tension'. Later, researchers changed to 'premenstrual syndrome' to take into account the collection of related physical symptoms.

Many women say they feel like a different person before their period. They can become intensely irritable and snappy with everyone: husband, kids, workmates, even the doctor or, worse, the boss. The forgetfulness and inability to focus attention that often accompany this make even the simplest tasks take much longer than they should – increasing the sense of frustration and being out of control. At other times, the mood is one of deep depression. Self-confidence flies out of the window. The sufferer may experience attacks of irrational panic or anxiety; she is no longer in control of her own emotions.

Another feature is that the risk of accidents while driving are increased. Hitting stationary objects through poor concentration or bad judgement, perhaps trying to squeeze too quickly into too small a space, is costly. Driving aggressively, perhaps overtaking without due care, can be lethal.

TENDER BREASTS

Even if someone just brushes accidentally against my breasts
I want to scream, they're so sore.

It is quite common for breasts to enlarge in the two weeks before a period, returning to normal after the period begins. Premenstrual breast pain (mastalgia) affects some five million women in Britain between the ages of twenty and fifty. It can affect part or all of the breast and even extend to the upper arms. Other benign (that is, non-cancerous) breast problems include nodularity, or lumpiness, in the breast just before a period.

Although women with breast pain appear to have normal hormone levels, their breast tissues are probably unusually sensitive to the actions of those hormones. This increased sensitivity is linked to the levels of essential fatty acids (EFAs) in the bloodstream, which could explain why the problem frequently responds to regular supplements of evening primrose oil, a source of the EFA gamma-linolenic acid (GLA). Sufferers may also have high blood levels of saturated fats, which can increase the effects of hormones on breast tissue. Painkillers and diuretics are frequently ineffective and may carry their own side-effects.

ABDOMINAL DISTENSION AND WEIGHT-GAIN

My stomach feels bloated out and my face looks puffy. If I can get my jeans on at all, they'll be too uncomfortable to wear anyway. When I start wearing my saggy old skirt with the elasticated waistband my husband says he knows exactly what's coming!

One of the most commonly reported symptoms, this can also be one of the most upsetting. Many women regularly report putting on several pounds overnight, waking up with a puffy face, swollen ankles and an uncomfortable, bloated abdomen. In fact, the weight-gain is just water retention, and it will almost certainly disappear as quickly as it came, shortly after the period starts. But finding your clothes are too tight is demoralising and, if you have been dieting, there is nothing worse than devoting three weeks of self-denial to losing five pounds, only to see as much weight climb back on in the space of twenty-four hours.

CLUMSINESS

It's as though my fingers and thumbs are all knitted together – I drop crockery, cigarettes, make stupid typing errors, cut myself.

Dropping things, forgetfulness, confusion: this is particularly distressing if you are in a job where you have to keep your mind sharp, because such symptoms can be mistaken for inability and incompetence. And attributing errors to PMS does you no good whatsoever – in a competitive world, being a slave to your hormones is hardly a career advantage! If you also suffer from tension premenstrually, then accidentally dropping a plate or losing your car keys can be guaranteed to take you to screaming point.

HEADACHES, SUGAR CRAVINGS AND LETHARGY

I was tired and I should've just gone to bed, but I just had to go back into the kitchen and there was half of the birthday cake left. I thought, just one slice, so I had one, then another, and ended up eating it all.

These three symptoms can all result from erratic swings in blood sugar levels. Snacking on sugary sweets or overdosing on caffeine can not only contribute to the cause, it can also compound the symptoms. For example, a sweet snack might boost energy levels temporarily, but will be followed by corresponding fatigue. You respond to that with another, similar snack ... and you could find yourself on a roller-coaster of activity and lethargy. Dietary strategies are particularly effective with these symptoms, and will be discussed fully in Chapter 4.

Types of PMS

A researcher in California, Dr Guy Abrahams, has identified four types of premenstrual syndrome, according to the groups of symptoms experienced, and he has attributed these symptoms to specific diet and lifestyle factors.

Type	Symptoms	Cause
PMS-A (anxiety)	Anxiety, panic attacks, nervous tension, mood swings, irritability	Deficiency of magnesium and Vitamin B6; excess caffeine intake
PMS-H (hydration)	Premenstrual weight-gain, abdominal bloating, water retention, breast tenderness	High salt or sugar intake; deficiencies of essential fatty acids

PMS-C (craving)	Food cravings, headaches, tiredness, dizziness, fainting	Excessive fluctuations in blood sugar levels; high caffeine intake
PMS-D (depression)	Depression, crying, forgetfulness, insomnia and confusion	Environmental factors; lack of exercise; excess weight; deficiencies in B vitamins, magnesium

His general advice includes attention to healthy eating, stress avoidance, cutting down on sweet foods and reducing cigarettes, coffee and alcohol.

Contributing Factors

There is no doubt that certain factors can make PMS symptoms worse:

* **Poor diet**, in particular, eating too much sugar and saturated fat. Indulging cravings for sweet, sugary foods can compound the problem by causing wild fluctuations in blood sugar levels, which can make you feel, by turns, shaky then tired, irritable then depressed.
* **Caffeine.** Chinese scientists found that there is a strong association between increased caffeine consumption and severity of premenstrual symptoms. Those women suffering most were also drinking most coffee. There could be a hormonal link here – we know that high oestrogen levels slow down the rate at which caffeine is broken down by the liver.
* **Essential fatty acid deficiency.** These are the raw materials from which hormones are made. If we are deficient in certain essential fatty acids, hormone production can be affected.

* **Obesity.** Excess fatty tissue has an effect on oestrogen production and so can affect the hormonal balance and increase the symptoms of PMS.
* **Drugs, alcohol and smoking.** Anything that has an effect on mood can, in turn, exacerbate the mood changes of PMS.
* **Pollution.** Many kinds of pollution can have an effect upon the availability of essential trace elements such as magnesium and zinc, which can influence hormone production.
* **Oral contraceptives.** These and other artificial sources of hormones can influence the body's hormone balance.
* **Stress.** Psychological and physical stress can influence the brain and the output of hormones from the pituitary gland, which controls the output of sex hormones.
* **Pregnancy.** Although the nine months of pregnancy usually render a women blissfully free of her regular symptoms, PMS sometimes get worse afterwards, particularly after a second pregnancy.
* ***Candida albicans***. The thrush-causing bacterial infection produces symptoms which can be mistaken for PMS. It can also exacerbate the effect of the syndrome itself. If you have a tendency to thrush, your PMS symptoms are likely to be worse.

——— 2 ———
Know Your Body

Monthly periods begin during the early to mid-teens and continue, albeit with interruptions, for thirty to forty years. During the earlier years, periods tend to be irregular, and it is not usually until the twenties that they settle down to a consistent pattern. This pattern is interrupted by pregnancies and breastfeeding, which bring about considerable hormonal upheaval, but the menstrual cycle naturally resumes.

Between the ages of forty and fifty-five, towards the end of a woman's fertile life, a degree of irregularity returns to the cycle. This heralds the start of the menopause and the end of the reproductive years.

PMS can be a problem at any stage between the very first period and the onset of the menopause. Some women will suffer throughout this time; others will not develop any symptoms at all until, perhaps, after having a couple of children. The only thing you can say with certainty about PMS is that the symptoms always coincide with the second half of the menstrual cycle, ie the few days before the period begins. To understand why, you need to know a little about the changes that take place in the body during the menstrual cycle.

The Menstrual Cycle

The menstrual cycle is the process that enables a woman to conceive a child. Once a month the lining of the uterus, or womb, becomes thicker and ready to receive and nourish a fertilised egg. If pregnancy does not result, the cycle ends with the shedding of the lining of the uterus – the discharge of bloody matter lasting for several days, which is called the menstrual period, or menstruation. After the period has ended and the lining has been shed, the uterus starts once more to build and thicken a new lining.

The length of the cycle varies for different women and will often fluctuate a little for an individual. Anything from twenty-two to thirty-five days from day one of your menstrual period to the first day of your next period is considered normal.

It is the process of menstruation that we are most conscious of, because we can actually see and feel the regular flow of blood. We may also suffer some pain. But inside our bodies there are other important events taking place right through the cycle, of which we are usually completely unaware.

The most significant event happens in the middle of the cycle, usually around fourteen days after the first day of your period. This is ovulation, when a ripe new egg bursts free from one of the ovaries. It is caught within the funnel-shaped opening of the end of the fallopian tube, and as it is wafted down this tube towards the uterus it may meet a sperm and be fertilised. While the egg travels, other subtle body changes take place which are designed to enhance the chances of the woman becoming pregnant. The cervix, ie the mouth of the womb, becomes softer and opens slightly to allow sperm to enter. Specialised cells in the cervix produce a clear, slippery mucus which is particularly nourishing and inviting to sperm.

If unprotected intercourse coincides with the days in which these conditions are prevalent, a pregnancy will more easily result. If it does not, the unfertilised egg is shed, along with the lining of the uterus, in the menstrual period.

The Role of Sex Hormones

The whole menstrual process is initiated every month by a gland in the brain called the pituitary. This tiny pea-shaped organ produces follicle-stimulating hormone (FSH) and luteinising hormone (LH). It is FSH that tells the ovary to produce a ripened egg. It is in response to FSH that the ovary in turn secretes the female sex hormone oestrogen. Oestrogen controls the first half of the cycle, and one of its roles is controlling the thickening of the uterus lining ready for pregnancy, which it does up to the point at which the egg leaves the ovary.

Once the oestrogen has reached a high enough level in the bloodstream, the ovary finally releases the ripe egg from the blister-like follicle that encloses it – around day fourteen. At this point, the pituitary gland stops producing FSH and produces LH instead.

The follicle that is left empty on the surface of the ovary now acquires a life of its own. It becomes known as the corpus luteum and it begins to produce a second sex hormone, progesterone. Progesterone helps to further thicken the lining of the uterus. If the egg is not fertilised, the corpus luteum becomes smaller and dies away around day twenty-two of the cycle, and the progesterone level in the blood falls. Finally, the uterus lining is shed around day twenty-eight in the menstrual period.

A further hormone, prolactin, is secreted by the pituitary. This is the hormone that stimulates the breasts to produce milk after childbirth. During the normal, non-pregnant, menstrual cycle prolactin seems to regulate the amounts of oestrogen and progesterone produced by the ovaries.

Severe physical or mental stress can actually cause the pituitary gland to bring the monthly action of the ovaries to a complete halt. For example, it is not unusual for female athletes to stop having periods altogether through the effect of regular high-level exercise on their hormones. For the rest of us, great emotional stress can cause our period to be late or missed altogether. For example, in students, examination stress has been found to alter the length of menstrual cycles. During an examination, a much higher proportion of the female population will be menstruating than you would expect on the basis of chance, which means that a proportion of the girls will have suffered PMS during revision time.

What Causes PMS?

Many theories have been put forward to explain the processes that cause individual PMS symptoms. Why exactly should we retain water at this time? Why should we become irritable, depressed, clumsy? The following sections outline a number of explanations which have been proposed, based on what we already know about the biochemistry of the female body. It is likely that the full story is a combination of these, along with other factors as yet undiscovered. The following, though, is useful in explaining particular symptoms as well as the logic behind, and the success of, certain treatment programmes.

HORMONES AND PMS

As well as controlling the physical changes that happen to a woman's body during the menstrual cycle, oestrogen and progesterone can also have an effect on mood. Oestrogen can act as a stimulant, resulting in anxiety, irritability and tension. Progesterone, on the other hand, is a depressant, so a correct balance between the two hormones throughout the cycle is important.

Too much prolactin from the pituitary gland can upset this balance. Diet and nutrition, exercise and stress, all seem to have their own influence upon this balance. Certain nutrients such as vitamin B6, vitamin C, zinc and magnesium play a special role.

True symptoms of premenstrual syndrome only occur in the second half of the menstrual cycle, which is when the ovaries are busiest producing female hormones. The fact that both oestrogen and progesterone are being produced in large quantities around the time that we experience PMS makes them the primary suspects. We also find that, when the ovaries are either removed surgically or have their action suppressed by drugs – removing the hormonal cycle – the symptoms of PMS usually disappear.

The obvious conclusion to make is that PMS is caused by the output of hormones from the ovaries. But it is not as simple as that. In fact, there is no evidence that women with PMS have abnormal levels of progesterone and oestrogen, or indeed any of the other hormones whose levels vary through the menstrual cycle.

Instead, experts now believe that the symptoms are caused by the way that the body handles the normal fluctuations in these

FEMALE SEX HORMONE ACTIVITY
THROUGH THE MENSTRUAL CYCLE

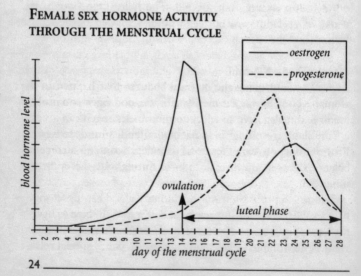

hormone levels. It seems it is normal ovarian function, rather than any hormone imbalance, that triggers the symptoms every month, and so the fault lies in the way we react to our own natural sex hormones.

BLOOD SUGAR LEVELS AND PMS

Mood changes and cravings premenstrually could be caused by the effect of sex hormones on blood sugar levels.

In healthy people, levels of the simple sugar, glucose, in the blood, are maintained within strict limits by hormones which operate as part of a highly efficient feedback mechanism. When blood glucose rises, the hormone insulin is released from the pancreas. Insulin causes some of the glucose to be removed from the blood by moving it into body cells to be burnt for energy, or to be converted into forms for longer term storage: to glycogen, a complex carbohydrate that is kept in the liver, or simply to fat.

It's a bit like the way you control the amount of food in your fridge. If it gets too full, you might take some food out to eat, and other foods you might put into the deep freeze to use another time.

Conversely, if blood glucose levels fall below a certain limit, secretion of a hormone called glucagon is triggered which causes glucose to be released from body stores. To continue the analogy, just as you defrost some of the food from your freezer and put it back into the fridge for imminent use.

If blood glucose falls to a dangerous level, another hormone, adrenaline, is released from the adrenals: two triangular glands that sit on the top of each kidney. Adrenaline gives a further boost to the process of converting liver glycogen back into glucose.

In PMS, it seems as though the lower limit of blood sugar is set too high, so that adrenaline is released earlier than it should be. Now, adrenaline doesn't just control blood sugar levels. It is also the hormone that is secreted in response to fear and crisis, and it orchestrates the body's response to danger, priming it for action. Think about the feelings you get when you are frightened: heart beating faster, nervous tension, anxiety, panic ... do those sound familiar? Where the same reactions happen in the body of a woman who is not confronted with danger or crisis, you can understand why she finds herself becoming aggressive, experiencing panic attacks or getting bad tempered or impatient. It seems that she is being made to experience normal feelings, caused by a healthy body reaction, but at the wrong time.

So why should premenstrual women be prone to releasing adrenaline at inappropriate times? The answer could be

THE EFFECT OF COMPLEX CARBOHYDRATES AND SIMPLE SUGARS ON BLOOD GLUCOSE LEVELS

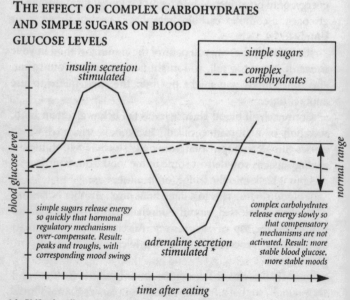

—— simple sugars

‑ ‑ ‑ complex carbohydrates

insulin secretion stimulated

blood glucose level

normal range

simple sugars release energy so quickly that hormonal regulatory mechanisms over-compensate. Result: peaks and troughs, with corresponding mood swings

adrenaline secretion stimulated *

complex carbohydrates release energy slowly so that compensatory mechanisms are not activated. Result: more stable blood glucose, more stable moods

time after eating

* *In PMS, adrenaline secretion may be stimulated even before blood glucose has dropped below the normal range, making control even more difficult.*

progesterone. As well as preparing the lining of the uterus, progesterone is also involved in regulating blood sugar levels – it plays a role in the lowering mechanism, so that if there is not enough progesterone circulating, the baseline for the lower level of blood sugar is raised. The result? Even with blood sugar levels within normal limits, surges of adrenaline may occur, producing those inappropriate and alarming mood symptoms.

Eating complex carbohydrates could help. Complex carbohydrates release energy into the body slowly, so that compensatory mechanisms are not activated. Result: more stable blood glucose; more stable moods.

On the other hand, simple sugars release energy so quickly that hormonal regulatory mechanisms over-compensate. Result: peaks and troughs of blood glucose levels, with corresponding mood swings.

PROLACTIN AND PMS

Prolactin is released by the pituitary gland into the bloodstream in pulses throughout the menstrual cycle, and its levels can be increased by stress or by stimulation of the breasts. High levels can limit the amount of progesterone released in the second half of the menstrual cycle, with the effects on blood sugar levels already described. High prolactin levels also seem to cause or worsen water-retention symptoms such as bloated abdomen and breast pain.

Some PMS sufferers do indeed have abnormally high levels of blood prolactin. Most, though, have normal levels. But there is evidence that deficiency of essential fatty acids (EFAs) can result in oversensitivity to these normal levels, so the woman suffers as if she had raised prolactin levels.

If we look closely at EFAs and how they are used in the body, it is possible to explain how they are implicated in PMS and understand why certain nutritional supplements could help with the symptoms.

EFAS AND PMS

Essential fatty acids are a small group of compounds found naturally in certain fats, and are vital for health. One, cis-linoleic acid, is the raw material for the production of a vital hormone-like chemical called prostaglandin E1 (PGE1). This is involved in a range of actions in the body including blood pressure control, insulin manufacture and inflammation reduction, and is also necessary for correct hormonal balance during the premenstrual period.

We cannot make cis-linoleic acid in the body – it has to be supplied through the diet. It comes from vegetable sources, of which the richest are oils such as sunflower, safflower and corn oil. Cooking and other forms of processing can affect the levels of cis-linoleic acid present in oils by converting it to forms that are less useful to the body, and that can even inhibit the process of PGE1 formation.

In the body, cis-linoleic acid is first converted to gamma-linolenic acid (GLA). This compound also happens to be found naturally in evening primrose oil, blackcurrant seed oil and borage oil, and may explain the effectiveness of these oils in relieving PMS symptoms in some women.

Even if you are getting plenty of cis-linoleic acid in your diet (and it is difficult to be deficient), you cannot guarantee you will be able to make all the GLA you need, because this initial reaction is vulnerable to being blocked by a number of factors. The enzyme that enables the conversion to take place can only function in the presence of adequate supplies of vitamin B6 (pyridoxine), zinc and magnesium, so these must be supplied by the diet. Its action is inhibited, on the other hand, by stress, advancing age, virus infections, alcohol consumption and a high-sugar or saturated-fat diet.

Once gamma-linolenic acid is formed in the body (or supplied externally) the next step is for it to be modified into a form called di-homo gamma-linolenic acid, and thence to

FACTORS AFFECTING THE CONVERSION OF CIS-LINOLEIC ACID TO PROSTAGLANDIN E1

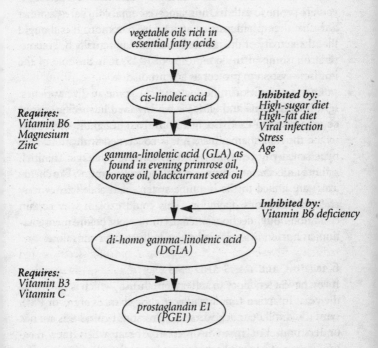

PGE1, this final reaction being subject to the availability of vitamins B3 and C.

It follows that anything that affects this chain of reactions – whether it be insufficient supply of the raw material, or inhibition of any of the enzymes that facilitate the chemical reactions, will reduce the amount of PGE1 produced. As a result, one becomes unusually sensitive to normal prolactin levels, and this can lead to PMS symptoms.

The Immune System and PMS

Any chronic illness tends to become worse before a period. If you are prone to asthma, migraines, eczema, cold sores, acne or arthritis, then premenstrual attacks are common. It is thought that the activity of the immune system may actually be responsible for some of the symptoms of PMS. It is the role of the immune system to protect us against disease.

Our antibodies (immunoglobulins) come in five varieties: IgA, IgD, IgE, IgG and IgM. Each is involved in specific actions or reactions. For example, IgA is involved in fighting infections in the mucous membranes; IgE is concerned with immediate hypersensitivity reactions, such as hayfever (allergic rhinitis), asthma and eczema. Some prostaglandins (hormone-like chemicals) are linked to the immune system, and a deficiency may affect the system's operation. This could explain why certain conditions and infections often occur or recur before menstruation, as hormone levels are known to fluctuate at this time.

CANDIDA ALBICANS AND PMS

If you have a tendency to suffer from thrush, which is caused by the yeast infection *Candida albicans,* the chances are your PMS symptoms will be much worse. The reasons behind this are not understood, but many women find that when they have brought yeast growth back under control their PMS symptoms become less severe.

Candida is normally present in small quantities in our intestines, where its growth is controlled by the presence of competing bacteria. Certain circumstances can alter the environment of the intestinal tract – pregnancy, a course of antibiotics, use of the oral contraceptive pill – so that the balance between the flora living there changes and the yeast cells multiply out of control.

Symptoms of *Candida* overgrowth include vaginal itching and discharge, digestive upsets such as constipation, diarrhoea or excessive wind and disturbances of the menstrual cycle, all of which can affect general mental well-being.

If *Candida* is suspected as a factor in PMS, it can be treated by antifungal drugs such as Nystatin, available on prescription. While you are being treated, you can help limit further yeast growth by changes in diet. Foods that are particularly attractive to *Candida* are those that are high in carbohydrates, and which contain yeast or which have been fermented. So you should avoid the following foods:

* sugary foods and sweets
* yeast-baked foods such as bread (use unleavened breads and crispbreads instead)
* wine, beer, cider and vinegar
* cheese (use only unfermented cheeses such as curd or cottage cheese)
* starchy vegetables such as potatoes and parsnips
* mushrooms.

FOOD ALLERGY AND PMS

Many specific food allergies can cause or exacerbate PMS symptoms. For advice on common food allergies, see Chapter 4. It is often the case that the foods that we crave the most actually cause the allergic reaction. So if you crave a lot of bread, try giving it up for a week – you may discover that it is the cause of your symptoms! The most common problem foods are yeast, wheat, dairy produce, citrus fruits and mushrooms. For more information about food allergies, see my *Quick Guide to Food Allergies*.

How to Tell

There are over 150 different symptoms associated with PMS, both physical and emotional, and they are so diverse that you might not be able immediately to identify them as part of the syndrome. If in doubt, see if the following criteria apply:

* symptoms must have occurred every month for at least the previous three months
* symptoms occur only in the second part of the menstrual cycle, ie during the days before a period
* symptoms disappear completely after the onset of the heaviest day of your period, and do not reappear for at least seven days.

No matter what the symptoms, the diagnosis of PMS is entirely dependent upon when they happen in relation to menstruation. The best method of diagnosis available today is the simple and inexpensive one of recording dates of menstruation and symptoms. This is good news for PMS sufferers, because it means your diagnosis is in your own hands. If you suspect that your problems are due to PMS, start charting now.

KEEP A RECORD

Charting your symptoms can help in more ways than one:

1 You can confirm that your problems really are related to your menstrual cycle. Just knowing the cause can be reassuring in itself, and it also helps you plan your life. If your periods are regular, and you can calculate ahead the dates that are likely to coincide with PMS, then you can avoid disastrous clashes. Peak time is not a good day to have the in-laws over for dinner, take your driving test, or make a major business presentation to a new client!

2 The type of symptoms recorded may help to point your doctor towards treatments that might be most effective. Groups of symptoms linked to water retention, for

example, would be approached differently from those resulting from fluctuations in blood sugar levels.

3 If you decide to seek your doctor's advice, a well-kept record of symptoms over the last three months or so will help him or her considerably in diagnosis. What is more, if your GP is unsympathetic or sceptical as to the existence of PMS, he or she is likely to be more understanding if you can show a methodical, reasoned approach to the problem than if you turn up at the surgery in a flood of tears or snarling irritably.

The National Association for Premenstrual Syndrome (NAPS) recommend using a chart similar to the one reproduced in Appendix 1 at the back of this book. You can copy this so that you have a chart of your own to write on.

Enter the days on which you are menstruating with an 'M' or use a red pen to draw a line through those days. Insert appropriate symbols to indicate the days of your most severe symptoms. I've suggested initial letters here – you can invent your own, perhaps choosing just your three main symptoms so that the chart is as clear as possible. Use a lower case letter if the symptom is mild, and a capital letter if it is severe. Get into the habit of filling in the chart at the same time every day, eg each night before you go to bed, so that you do not forget. It is a good idea to keep an accurate record for three months, or more, before showing your doctor, because it usually takes at least this long to identify a clear and consistent pattern, unfortunately.

If your moods – temper, irritability, depression – are particularly troublesome, why not give a second chart to your partner, or someone with whom you have close contact day to day? Their independent assessment of your mood will be valuable and it should be interesting to compare the two charts.

If three months of diligent charting confirms that symptoms do occur only in the fourteen days before menstruation, and are absent for at least seven days after your period starts, then you have met the criteria for having PMS.

3

PMS Remedies

For some women, it is enough to provide simple reassurance, an opportunity to discuss their problems with other sufferers, and perhaps some counselling to make their monthly symptoms manageable. For others, self-help measures such as change of diet, cutting out coffee and alcohol, or relaxation exercises will be sufficient. Most self-help treatments are free of charge, have no side-effects, and are likely to improve your general health anyway, which is never a bad thing! Increasing your health and general self-esteem could also improve your body's tolerance to the changes that take place premenstrually. So it is a good idea to try the simple, and cheap, DIY remedies before consulting your GP.

According to a recent survey of nearly 300 GPs carried out by the Women's Nutritional Advisory Service, half the doctors expressed difficulty in treating PMS. Although many now recognise that nutrition could be, to a large extent, responsible for the symptoms of PMS in many of their patients, and that the symptoms may be considerably relieved by changes in eating habits, very few GPs are confident in their ability to offer suitable dietary advice to women with PMS. In fact, 92 percent admitted to having no nutritional training whatsoever.

Because your doctor may well not be fully aware of the type of dietary changes that could help relieve your symptoms, you would be well advised to try self-help in the form of the eating plans detailed in Chapters 4 and 5.

An interesting fact to bear in mind is that, in studies of various treatments, a high placebo effect is evident. This means that, when women are given a 'dummy' treatment and told it may relieve their symptoms, in at least 50 percent the dummy treatment will work, even though there is no medical reason why it should. This perhaps demonstrates the power of reassurance – knowing that the problem is being taken seriously – in bringing relief.

What to Expect from Your GP

You cannot be tested for PMS. There is no physical examination your doctor can do to confirm what is wrong. He or she won't be able to dip a stick into a bottle of your urine, or send a blood sample off to a laboratory to obtain a conclusive diagnosis. And, as we have already seen, there are no classic symptoms that can be used to identify the presence of PMS beyond doubt. So, the most reliable information you can present your GP with is your chart showing the symptoms experienced at different times of your menstrual cycle.

Once your GP has had the opportunity to examine your chart and confirm that the symptoms are indeed due to PMS, he or she should also examine you to rule out other gynaecological conditions that could be exacerbating your problems, such as endometriosis, an ovarian cyst or thyroid disease.

In women, the symptoms of depression are sometimes mistaken for PMS, and likewise PMS can be misdiagnosed as depression if the cyclical nature of the symptoms has not been spotted. So it may also be necessary to eliminate the possibility of a psychiatric disorder, especially if your symptoms do not have a clear-cut cyclical pattern.

You may also be given a questionnaire with which to record details of your normal diet. This will include space for noting things like alcohol, tobacco, tea and coffee consumption, use of salt with food, and your normal meal and snacking patterns.

Where symptoms are severe, a specialist may choose to undertake what is known as a 'gonadotrophin releasing hormone analogue test'. This involves a monthly dose of a compound which completely suppresses the cyclical activity of the ovaries. It is carried out for three months and the patient is asked to monitor the effect on symptoms. If they are eliminated, then it is fair to assume that the symptoms depend upon the activity of the ovaries, ie this is true PMS.

Treatments for PMS

The following includes details of both conventional and alternative remedies for PMS. All of the treatments mentioned here have been effective for some women, but there is no one remedy that has ever been shown to work for all. Until the causes of PMS are properly understood, it is be impossible to give any woman a guarantee that a particular treatment might work for her. All you can do is try different treatment strategies, noting their effects on your symptom chart, until you come to one – or even a combination of treatments – that seems to alleviate your symptoms.

NON-MEDICAL THERAPIES

The use of supplements of vitamin B6, calcium and magnesium has some theoretical basis. All are involved in the process of manufacturing neurotransmitters: chemicals involved in the body's communications system. Clinical trials of individual nutrients have been carried out to investigate the effectiveness of these supplements further, but so far results do not agree – some support their use; others do not.

Evening Primrose Oil

Evening primrose oil is now the most solidly researched, as well as the simplest, approach to treating PMS. It has been tested in dozens of clinical trials, including many placebo-controlled studies. In this type of study, a drug's efficacy is compared to that of a dummy (or placebo) treatment which is given to patients who are unaware of whether they are getting the real thing or not. Such trials are able to test whether the effect of the drug is purely psychological. It seems that, with evening primrose oil, there is a good chance that in a great many women it is not.

As well as achieving a good success rate in relieving symptoms of PMS, trials have shown that the beneficial response to treatment seems to be sustained indefinitely so as long as you keep taking it. Another good feature of this treatment is that tolerance does not seem to develop: this is where the treatment becomes less effective with time and the patient has to take ever-increasing doses to achieve the same relief.

Evening primrose oil is a good source of gamma-linolenic acid (GLA), and it is believed to be this ingredient that is active in relieving PMS symptoms. Other rich sources of GLA include blackcurrant seed oil, starflower oil and borage oil, and although these have not received the same level of attention from scientists, they may also be effective. There are a great number of products on the market containing these ingredients, and most are quite costly, so you may find it is worth taking a calculator with you to the health-food shop to find which products give you the best value!

If you are planning to try evening primrose oil, you should be prepared to persist with taking at least 500mg every day throughout the menstrual cycle for three to six months before deciding whether or not it works for you. Many experts recommend much larger amounts, between 3,000 and 4,000mg a day. As the oil works by gradually changing the essential fatty acid composition of cell membranes it is inevitably a slow cure, so you are unlikely to notice any effect within the first couple of months.

In one trial carried out at St Thomas's Hospital in London, sixty-eight women whose PMS symptoms had failed to respond to conventional treatments were given 2,000mg evening primrose oil a day. Sixty-one percent reported total relief from PMS, and a further 23 percent found partial relief. Another trial involving eighty-nine patients compared the effect of 500mg per day evening primrose oil with that of a placebo. Those taking the evening primrose oil showed a marked improvement in symptoms over those given the placebo.

Premenstrual breast tenderness responds well to treatment with evening primrose oil, and patients suffering from mastalgia (severe breast pain) can now obtain the oil on prescription in a form called Efamast. Evening primrose oil is one of the few natural products to receive a medical licence (it can also be obtained on prescription for eczema).

At the University of Wales Breast Clinic a clinical trial found that 45 percent of women who had persistent, severe breast pain benefited from a 3,000mg per day dose of evening primrose oil. The treatment was as effective as the commonly prescribed drugs bromocriptine and danazole, but without the high levels of side-effects normally associated with the drugs. The medical team reported in *The Lancet* that, after ruling out the possibility of cancer, evening primrose oil should be the first line of treatment for breast pain.

Note: Evening primrose oil is not suitable if you are epileptic, as it can sometimes make this condition worse.

Vitamin B6 (Pyridoxine)

Vitamin B6, often a first-line nutritional treatment, is believed to influence hormone action by helping the body make more efficient use of available EFAs. So, if your diet is low in EFAs, with the result that your body becomes oversensitive to the action of the hormone prolactin (as explained in Chapter 2), vitamin B6 can reduce the severity of symptoms, particularly breast tenderness, by helping you use what supply of EFA you do have to the best possible advantage.

The recommended daily allowance of vitamin B6 is 2mg per day, and most people get enough from meat, fish, cereals and vegetables. But it is possible that some women do not absorb it well from their food. Supplements, prescribed in quantities of 100–200mg per day taken throughout the cycle, can alleviate symptoms in some women. It may take three months before the benefits of B6 start to show, but it's worth persevering. In one trial, vitamin B6 at a daily dosage of 40–100mg was found effective in 50–60 percent of a group of seventy PMS patients.

Note: Larger doses, taken for prolonged periods of time, may cause the condition known as peripheral neuropathy, symptoms of which include 'pins and needles', numbness and painful burning sensations in the limbs. This can lead ultimately to nerve damage. If you are planning on buying over-the-counter B6 supplements, seek your GP's advice first on a dose that is likely to be safe, as well as effective, for you.

Vitamin E

This vitamin, which, among other things, influences the way we metabolise fats, has been shown to be effective for some symptoms at doses of between 150 and 600mg a day. Sufferers of depression and anxiety symptoms seem to derive the most benefit. Interestingly, the mineral selenium has synergistic effects in the body with vitamin E, so by taking selenium as well you should need less vitamin E. There are a number of supplements available that contain both nutrients, including a number that are sold as antioxidants for their general health benefits. Evening primrose oil capsules usually contain vitamin E.

Mineral Supplements

Modern diets and lifestyle factors may be reducing the amount of minerals that we absorb even if we seem to eat enough in our food. For example, magnesium is believed to be lowered by levels of fluoride in drinking water. Zinc is thought to be lowered by the contraceptive pill, refined carbohydrates (such as white flour and sugar), alcohol, smoking, some food additives and by the body having to fight infection or heal wounds. Chromium levels can be affected by too much sugar and alcohol.

What is more, diets that are high in roughage, such as bran, can also reduce your ability to absorb essential minerals. Bran and other insoluble fibres can absorb water and certain minerals like a sponge, carrying them through the digestive system to be passed straight out of the body again. So it is not wise to sprinkle bran onto meals in the belief that you are making your diet healthier. A better way to step up your fibre intake is to eat more fresh fruit and vegetables, beans and pulses, and switch to wholemeal cereal products.

Never exceed the dose of either medically prescribed mineral supplements, or that given on proprietary brands of mineral preparations. It is possible to overdose on some minerals, and increasing the amount of one mineral sometimes interferes with the body's use of another.

These are the minerals most commonly associated with PMS:

Magnesium. Some, but not all, PMS sufferers have reduced levels of the mineral magnesium in their red blood cells. Conversely, not all women with low blood cell magnesium suffer from PMS. We don't yet know what part magnesium might play in PMS, but there is some evidence that correcting low magnesium levels relieves symptoms in some women. This is important when you realise that around 15 percent of women in the UK are probably not getting enough of this essential mineral. Good food sources are nuts, wholegrain cereals, meat and fish.

Zinc. Around one woman in twenty does not get enough zinc in her daily diet. Zinc's roles in the body include hormone production, as well as maintaining the immune system and keeping skin healthy. It is found in meat, seafood (especially oysters), yeast and eggs.

Chromium. Though not strictly classed as an essential mineral, a growing number of experts believe that an adequate intake of chromium is vital for health. In particular, it seems to be important in the control of blood sugar levels through its action on the hormone insulin. Increasing age, and a too-high intake of sugary or refined foods, is believed to increase chromium loss from the body. You can step up your intake by eating more yeast-containing foods, liver and wholegrain cereals.

In the above, one has to remember the potential problems with yeast infections and food allergies as some foods make these conditions worse.

MEDICAL THERAPIES

If PMS symptoms are so severe that they interfere with normal family life or work, and where there are serious relationship problems or a risk of assault, self-injury or alcohol abuse, then doctors will generally turn to drug therapy. Which drug depends on the patient. Older women, who are close to the menopause, are the best candidates for treatment with the hormone oestrogen because it suppresses ovulation, and would not therefore be suitable for a young woman who may wish to become pregnant.

As with all medications, care must be taken during pregnancy, so always let your GP know if there is any chance you may become pregnant during treatment. Some preparations may harm a developing foetus.

In very severe cases, surgery may be performed as a last resort. Removal of the uterus and ovaries is probably the only permanent cure for PMS, but this is used very rarely and is obviously a drastic measure.

Progesterone

Despite the fact that progesterone has been used widely for many years, experts still argue over how valuable it really is in treating PMS. There is a great deal of anecdotal evidence as to its efficacy and it is widely promoted by many experts with enthusiasm, but its performance in clinical trials has not so far been conclusive.

Progesterone preparations contain the hormone identical to that found naturally in a woman's body, with the active ingredient made from a compound isolated from soya beans. It cannot be given in tablet form, as the hormone would be digested and metabolised by the liver before it ever reached the receptor sites. Progesterone is therefore given either in the form of pessaries which are inserted into the rectum or vagina (eg Cyclogest), or as an injection into the buttock (eg Gestone), where the hormone readily dissolves in the fat cells there. Symptoms should improve within an hour or so, whichever treatment is used.

Treatment, which is given daily, begins each month at the time of ovulation, about half-way through the menstrual cycle, and continues until the full flow of menstruation. If treatment begins before ovulation has taken place, it may have the effect of shortening the cycle. The dosage required by each individual to keep her symptoms under control varies widely, so in the early stages adjustments should be made to find the optimum level.

Progesterone seems to have a wide safety margin and side-effects are rare. Neither is it believed to react with other medications that a patient may be taking at the same time for different conditions. For comparison, during pregnancy, blood levels of progesterone can reach 30–50 times the levels found during a normal menstrual cycle – progesterone treatment for PMS is unlikely to raise levels to this degree.

It is a good idea to continue monitoring your symptoms on your menstrual chart, so that your GP can track the success of the treatment and any slight changes in the pattern of menstruation.

Progestogens (Synthetic Progesterone)

Progestogens (Duphaston or Primolut N) are synthetic versions of the hormone progesterone. The drug can be taken in the form of tablets, or sometimes is injected, and it takes three months before benefits start to show. Although progestogens do work for many women, experts believe they are less likely than natural progesterone to reach the widespread and specific receptor sites and thereby raise plasma progesterone levels. In some cases, progestogens can even make the symptoms of PMS worse. Because progestogens can be effective at treating heavy, painful or too-frequent periods, they may be best reserved for women whose PMS is also associated with these symptoms.

Oral Contraceptives

The combined contraceptive pill is sometimes prescribed to relieve symptoms of PMS. The oestrogen in the pill disturbs the menstrual cycle so that the woman's body does not enter the second half of the cycle, which is when PMS symptoms occur. In theory, then, it should be effective. In practice, the evidence to support their use is limited.

All oral contraceptives contain the synthetic hormone progestogen and this can sometimes make PMS worse, as it depresses the level of natural progesterone in the blood. In fact, some non-sufferers have actually reported developing symptoms of PMS when they start taking the pill!

Oestrogen is not usually given alone because it has been associated with a slight increase in the risk of cancer of the womb.

Oestrogen Patches

A newer treatment, which looks promising according to initial reports, is based on giving oestrogen in large doses by the use of stick-on skin patches similar to those used to help smokers kick their habit. Unlike the oestrogen used in the contraceptive pill, which is a synthetic form, the patches contain natural oestrogen in quite high doses, which is released slowly. This prevents ovulation from taking place, so the second phase of the cycle and the PMS symptoms associated with it should not arise.

As with the contraceptive pill, it is necessary for some progestogen to be given so that you continue to have a monthly bleed, and to guard against the slightly increased risk of cancer of the uterus. According to early studies, the progestogen dose does not seem to stimulate PMS symptoms (as it often does with the contraceptive pill), although in a long-term study in which women were treated over two to eight years with oestrogen patches and progestogen, almost six in ten developed new PMS symptoms – adjustments to the dose helped manage these problems.

Because ovulation does not take place, this treatment is best suited to women approaching the menopause.

Danazole
This drug can be used to block the action of the female sex hormones and so suppress ovulation – by doing this it removes the symptoms of PMS. Even in smaller doses, it can help reduce the symptoms. It can produce side-effects such as hair growth and deepening of the voice, although these changes are rare and reversible once the treatment is stopped. If pregnancy occurs during treatment there is a possibility of risk to the foetus.

Bromocriptine
Another powerful drug, bromocriptine blocks the action of the hormone prolactin, which is secreted by the pituitary gland and which acts on the breasts. It can be useful for severe breast tenderness, but is not a suitable option for long-term treatment.

Diuretics (Water Tablets)

These can be helpful as a short-term measure for relieving the discomforts of premenstrual water retention, such as weight-gain, abdominal bloating and breast tenderness. They are not, however, a long-term solution and cannot be expected to deal with any symptom that is not a direct result of water retention. Primary side-effects are thirst and potassium deficiency.

Mefenamic Acid (Ponstan)

This is a painkiller and anti-inflammatory drug of the NSAID group, sometimes prescribed for painful periods, which can also help relieve some premenstrual symptoms such as pelvic pain or headache.

TREATMENT OF *CANDIDA ALBICANS*

As explained in Chapter 2, PMS symptoms are often exacerbated by infection with the yeast *Candida albicans*, which produces thrush. If this is present, your GP can usually treat it with a course of fungicidal medication such as Nystatin. You can also help rebalance your intestinal flora by cutting down on sugary foods and yeast-containing foods (such as bread) and eating more natural yoghurt, especially those yoghurts which contain live acidophilus culture ('Bio' yoghurts).

HERBAL TREATMENTS

There are a number of herbal treatments that act as diuretics, ie they stimulate the kidneys to pass excess water. Herbs which are believed to have a natural diuretic effect include dandelion, fennel, parsley, raspberry leaf and yarrow. Usually, these are taken in the form of leaf tea. Other herbs can have a mild painkilling or tranquillising effect, as well as being recommended for depression, infections and inflammations. Ask at any good health-food shop about what is available.

ALTERNATIVE THERAPIES

Acupuncture, homoeopathy, reflexology, aromatherapy and massage have all been offered as treatments for PMS and some women do find them helpful, although they have not been studied scientifically. Reliable practitioners usually belong to a professional organisation and details are often available from public libraries or your local Citizens Advice Bureau. Alternatively, contact the Institute for Complementary Medicine (see Useful Addresses) for information on alternative therapies and local reputable practitioners.

When considering private alternative therapies and treatments, bear in mind that you may be vulnerable to pedlars of 'quack' cures. It is tempting to believe that every new treatment will be the solution to your problems, but if the suppliers of a product or treatment claim to offer a *guaranteed* cure for PMS, then you can bet that they cannot fulfil that claim.

If you are thinking of trying any new and expensive alternative treatment, check with your doctor first, or speak to somebody who has experience in dealing with PMS on one of the helplines given at the back of this book. If the treatment is authentic, then the chances are that these reputable organisations will already be aware of it and will be able to advise on whether it could help you.

WAYS TO HELP YOURSELF

No one remedy works for everyone, but there are lots of things you can try that cost you nothing, or next to nothing. The following ideas are all harmless and, if anything, might well improve your general health, which will at the very least help you to better tolerate your PMS symptoms.

Diet

Change to a low-fat, wholefood diet (further details are in Chapter 4).

REDUCE YOUR STRESS LEVELS

It is often possible to reduce stress premenstrually by planning ahead. Think about the situations in which you get most tense, eg if being stuck in traffic jams drives you mad, could you travel at a different time or take the train instead? What about all the time you spend at work trying to fix a jammed photocopier? You could promise yourself that next time it happens, if you haven't sorted the problem out within, say, ten minutes, you will stop and call the engineer. If meal preparation is fraught, cook ahead and freeze meals, cutting down time spent in the kitchen on bad days; or just get a takeaway. Work out strategies with the family, so they know there are certain times when you really need to be left alone.

Counselling

Ask at your local health centre if they have access to a trained counsellor – many do. Being able to talk over the difficulties caused by your changing moods can be extremely helpful.

Share the Experience

Many women find that it helps just to know they are not alone. Talk to your female friends, mother, sisters or daughters and share experiences. Make a pact with fellow sufferers to telephone each other at difficult times. Sometimes, only someone who has been through it can help you. Remember, too, that laughter is a great tension reliever, so an understanding friend who can make you see the funny side of your symptoms is a real gem.

There are also some useful helpline numbers given at the end of this book.

Exercise

Start a programme of regular activity. Don't make the mistake of overdoing it at the beginning or else you will probably never try to exercise again! Instead, spend time finding an activity you really enjoy, such as swimming, walking the dog, joining an aerobics class or following an exercise video in the privacy of your own home. Start off gradually and build up until you are exercising for about twenty minutes, three or four times a week. Don't exhaust yourself; find a pace that gets you warmed up and makes you breathe more deeply, but that you can manage without having to keep stopping for a rest. If you're pushed for time, or find classes and equipment too expensive, try to incorporate exercise into an everyday activity – walk the kids to school instead of driving them, for example.

Relaxation

A number of recent studies have found that relaxation techniques can be useful in relieving symptoms of PMS, and it seems as though they might be most effective in women whose symptoms are the most severe.

It is clear that the psychological trauma of PMS is made worse by the physical symptoms, and vice versa. For example, if your co-ordination is affected, you might drop and smash your best crockery; this will give you a shock and increase your stress levels, which in turn makes you more likely to scream at the children, and so on. Obviously, taking time out to relax will help to break the vicious circle.

Listen to your favourite soothing music, lying alone in a darkened room. Or try this: issue instructions that you must not be disturbed, then sink into a comfortable chair – with your feet up if you can – and close your eyes. Concentrate on your toes and curl them as tightly as you can for a second or two, as though you are trying to reach the sole of your foot. Now relax them completely. Think about your feet, tense the muscles for a couple of seconds, then let them, too, go limp. Next, do the same thing with your ankles, then your calves. Move up gradually through your whole body, tensing then relaxing, ending with the muscles of your neck, face and scalp. Then lie still for a few minutes, and recall pleasant memories, or imagine an idyllic scene. The whole process should take about fifteen minutes and leave you feeling very limp and relaxed. You may even fall asleep!

Appendix 2 at the back of this book shows a 'plan of action' for treatment of PMS, and could be used in conjunction with your chart of symptoms (Appendix 1). You may want to copy this for quick reference. It is not, however, a definitive guide –and the more drastic treatments will have to be discussed with your GP.

—4—

The PMS Diet

How Diet can Help

As we have already seen, although the causes of PMS are many and varied, the severity of the symptoms is to some extent under the woman's control, and choice of food and drink can play a large part.

It seems likely that PMS symptoms will be most troublesome when the following conditions apply:

* Blood sugar slips below the level that triggers the release of hormones that could affect moods (note that the premenstrual woman does not suffer from hypoglycaemia in the medical sense; rather, her set point is altered so that normal hormonal reactions to low blood sugar are triggered at levels that would be tolerated in non-sufferers).
* The diet lacks the vitamins, minerals, or EFAs needed for the chemical processes in the body that maintain correct hormonal balance.
* Too much salt is eaten – implicated in fluid retention.
* The diet is high in sugary foods, which exacerbate swings in blood sugar levels.
* There is high consumption of stimulants, such as: caffeine in coffee and, to a lesser extent, in tea; chocolate and cola drinks; alcohol and nicotine.
* There is an undiagnosed overgrowth of the yeast *Candida albicans*.

If these can be remedied by adopting a healthier diet, and if steps are taken to minimise stress and gently boost physical activity levels as well, the sufferer can often relieve symptoms considerably. For many women, this is enough to eliminate the need for medical help.

The Principles of a PMS Diet

It is as well to adopt the following principles permanently – not just for the premenstrual time. You should end up eating more healthily overall, and a fitter body is better able to withstand the effects of any challenge, whether it be physical, mental or hormonal.

The cornerstone of your PMS diet should be to ensure a regular intake of complex carbohydrates and a good supply of fibre. This helps to normalise blood sugar levels and so reduce the incidence of the mood swings and food cravings that can occur around this time.

Eating more frequently is important to keep blood sugar levels in check. Try not to go for more than three hours without at least a snack, and make sure all of your meals and snacks contain complex carbohydrate foods. This need not mean gaining weight. You can avoid increasing your total calorie intake simply by taking smaller meals with suitable snacks in between.

Your daily meal pattern could go something like this:

7.30am	Breakfast
10.30am	Mid-morning snack
1pm	Lunch
4pm	Afternoon snack
7pm	Dinner
10pm	Bedtime snack

There are no rigid rules over when you must eat – you can adjust the meal-times above to suit your own particular lifestyle – the important thing is to be sure that you never go too long without eating.

The Food Groups

The best way to get all the nutrition you need is to eat a good variety of foods every day. It helps to know what the different types of foods are, so you can balance your diet. If you eat a healthy balance of carbohydrates, proteins and fats every day, including plenty of fresh fruit and vegetables, then you should get all the vitamins and minerals you need.

CARBOHYDRATES
For our purposes, there are two types of carbohydrate – one is essential for your PMS diet, the other should be avoided.

Simple sugars are the PMS sufferer's arch enemy. These are easily digested and quickly absorbed into the bloodstream, where they send your blood glucose levels shooting up, until the body's compensatory mechanisms step in and bring them plummeting down again. When our blood glucose levels are low, we lack energy and often fall victim to food cravings. It is when levels are falling that PMS symptoms may be triggered.

Avoid foods rich in simple sugars. As well as cutting back on packet sugar, you should stay clear of all kinds of sweets and chocolates, biscuits, fizzy drinks (except the diet variety), cakes, honey, dried fruit and any processed food that includes large amounts of sugar or glucose syrup. Look at the label – the higher up in the list of ingredients, the more sugar in the food.

Complex carbohydrates, on the other hand, are your friends. Chemically, these are made up of long chains of simple sugars and, like them, complex carbohydrates are a source of energy. The difference is that complex carbohydrates take much longer to break down and be absorbed into the bloodstream. While they are being digested, the breakdown products gradually filter into the system over a sustained period of time – you receive your energy in a slow-release form – so blood sugar levels change gently and gradually and the peaks and troughs, which can be so disastrous in PMS sufferers, are avoided.

Complex carbohydrates include starchy foods such as bread, rice, pasta, potatoes, pulses and cereals. If there's a choice, opt for wholemeal cereal products, or brown (rather than white) rice for extra fibre, which keeps you feeling full for a little longer, further delaying the next snack attack. Wholegrain products are also much healthier foods in general. Many complex carbohydrate foods are also good sources of protein and B-vitamins, as well as being cheap and filling. Bananas come under this category because they are high in starch and they make a nutritious and filling snack.

Note: *Candida* sufferers must keep a check on their intake of carbohydrates, and especially those containing yeast (such as bread). Their dietary needs are discussed later.

PROTEIN
Protein is the substance of muscle and major body organs and is a constituent of every cell. Cells are constantly being broken down and replaced, so you need a good supply of protein foods every day to provide for ongoing growth and repair.

Meat, poultry, fish, eggs, dairy products, nuts and pulses (peas, beans and lentils) are all sources of protein. If you are a vegetarian, you should aim to get your protein from a variety of different sources, as plant proteins vary in their biological value. Milk, yoghurt and cheese are all good for you, but can be rich in fat, so if there's any worry about your weight, opt for lower-fat versions.

There is no particular value in eating a high-protein diet, as any excess is automatically converted into glucose and used for energy or stored as fat. Around 60g a day is an adequate intake for most women.

FATS

Fat is a highly concentrated source of energy, and it is the form in which we store our reserve supplies of energy. If we eat more calories than we need, whether they be from carbohydrate, protein or fat, they will end up stored in the form of fat.

There are many different types of fats, and for our purposes we should distinguish between the polyunsaturated fats (some of which contain the EFA cis-linoleic acid) and the saturated fats.

Polyunsaturated fats are found in many vegetable oils, such as corn oil, sunflower oil, safflower oil, and in margarines. These oils contain cis-linoleic acid. As explained in Chapter 2, inadequate supply of cis-linoleic acid can limit the production of prostaglandin E1, which is necessary for normal hormone function.

Saturated fats are found in animal fats such as butter, milk, cheese, and the fat in meats and meat products.

According to government guidelines, no more than 35 percent of your daily energy intake should be fat, and to ensure adequate intake of EFAs, around 6 percent of our total energy should be from the polyunsaturated varieties.

Ten-point Plan

1 **Cut down on simple sugars**

2 **Reduce fats, particularly saturated fats**

    ✱ Spread fats thinly on bread.

* If you must fry, use good quality sunflower, safflower and olive oils as these supply EFAs. Olive oil is best for cooking as it is the most stable at high temperatures. These oils are also excellent for making salad dressings.

3 Try to use less salt

* Add less salt to your cooking.
* Get out of the habit of automatically sprinkling salt onto your food at the table. Try the food first, then add a little salt only if it needs it.

4 Limit alcohol

* Alcohol can cause a sudden lowering of the blood sugar, which can lead to craving a sugary snack, so try to cut down on booze premenstrually.

5 Drink less coffee and tea

* Both contain caffeine which can aggravate anxiety and increase the risk of migraines.

6 Have complex carbohydrates with every meal and snack

* Slice of bread
* Couple of crispbreads
* Rice cakes
* Bowl of breakfast cereal
* Portion of cooked brown rice
* Small tin of baked beans
* Banana
* Jacket potato.

7 Eat frequently

* Don't go for more than three hours without a meal or snack.

8 Eat at least five servings of fresh produce a day

* This could be made up of a couple of pieces of fruit and three helpings of vegetables.
* If you don't have time to prepare and cook traditional vegetables with every meal then use them for your nibbles. Keep a bowl of juicy red tomatoes, or chunks of carrot floating in water, in the fridge; and a jar containing scrubbed sticks of green celery standing in water on the kitchen table.

9 Control your weight

* Resist the urge to indulge in chocolate and cakes when you are feeling premenstrual, as this will not only reduce your energy levels, it may also make you put on weight. Those who are overweight tend to have less energy than the rest of us, and the excess weight can itself be a cause of depression.

10 Make your new eating plan a lifetime habit

* The diet guidelines outlined in this *Quick Guide* will ensure that energy levels never fall and that you need not deprive your body of food to maintain a healthy weight. If you adopt this diet in the long term, the symptoms of PMS should decrease, hunger pangs will be banished and you will be getting all the nutrients you need to protect you against disease.

Candida

Those who suffer from *Candida albicans* infection (thrush), can help to keep the condition under control by avoiding certain foods and increasing the intake of others. Thrush is a very uncomfortable and frustrating condition that can make PMS symptoms more severe. Some people suffer from thrush throughout their lives, often as a result of something that they eat regularly.

Certain foods are thought to lead to the build-up of yeast that is responsible for thrush and avoiding these foods can make a real difference. Sweet foods should be avoided, including the more healthy varieties such as molasses and maple syrup. Small amounts of artificial sweeteners, such as aspartame, may be used as a substitute for sugar. Foods containing yeast should also be avoided, such as bread, Marmite, wines, beer, cider and other fermented beverages. Look carefully on food labels for yeast, as it is present in small amounts in a wide variety of processed foods. Yeast is also often added to vitamin supplements, so look out for this. As an alternative to bread, use unleavened breads and rye crispbreads, or you could bake your own using baking powder instead of yeast.

In general, foods that are fermented should be avoided. This includes the majority of cheeses, although cottage or ricotta cheese, which are made by curdling, can be eaten. All vinegars should also be avoided and lemon juice can be used in their place. Cut down on non-herbal teas – fortunately, there are a wide variety of delicious herbal teas available. Fruits, nuts and mushrooms are also thought to trigger *Candida*, so these should also be avoided. However, if you are not eating fruit, you should increase your intake of raw vegetables by snacking on carrots and celery and making sure that you have a salad or a couple of portions of cooked vegetables with every meal. It may also be a good idea to take an antioxidant supplement containing the

most important nutrients found in fresh fruit: beta-carotene
(vitamin A) and vitamin C.

Dietary Advice for
Specific PMS Symptoms

Abdominal bloating

Try cutting out coffee, tea, alcohol, sugar, yeast, dairy products,
wheat, oats, barley and rye. This may be a tall order, but after
you have cut out all of these foods, you can gradually reintro-
duce them to see if they are responsible for the bloating.

Cut down on salt; look carefully on all labels of processed
foods and don't add extra salt to your meals. Also cut down on
sugar and refined carbohydrates, such as white bread, pasta and
white rice, as these can aggravate the problem. A healthy diet
that is low in animal fats and rich in fruit and vegetables is best.

Anxiety and irritability

Avoid completely all drinks containing caffeine. This will
include coffee, tea and many fizzy drinks – scrutinise the list of
ingredients closely before you buy. Limit alcohol intake strictly,
and make sure you take frequent, regular meals containing
some protein.

Breast tenderness

A diet that is low in fat, high in protein and high in complex
carbohydrates is a good starting point here. Cut down on
caffeine and cigarettes.

Clumsiness

The connection between diet and clumsiness is not very clear,
but lack of certain nutrients and too much tea, coffee, cigarettes,
alcohol and other stimulants may be involved.

Depression
Cut down on junk foods, sweet foods and caffeine and omit all foods containing yeast. Also cut down on salt, dairy produce and alcohol.

Food cravings
The best way to keep hunger pangs and food cravings at bay is to eat regularly throughout the day. Make sure that you eat a complex carbohydrate at every meal and with snacks, as this will keep blood sugar levels stable. Avoid sweet foods, no matter how much you crave them, because as soon as you eat them, you will crave more, causing a Yo-Yo effect. Also steer clear of stimulants such as tea, coffee, cola, chocolate, alcohol and cigarettes.

Insomnia
Avoid all drinks containing caffeine, such as tea, coffee and cola, as these may keep you awake. It is also a good idea to have something light to eat just before you go to bed. A small amount of concentrated carbohydrate is ideal, such as a piece of toast or a couple of rice cakes. Do not eat cheese just before going to bed as it is difficult to digest. Alternatively, have some fruit, vegetables or yoghurt.

Migraine
Avoid cheese, chocolate, wine, tea, coffee, oranges, tomatoes and yeast-rich foods, including bread and Marmite.

—— 5 ——
High Energy Recipes

This final chapter puts the principles of the PMS diet into practice. Most of the recipes contain healthy forms of complex carbohydrates, which give us the energy to survive the day without feeling the need to snack on sweet foods. I have also included basic recipe ideas for cooking without yeast and sugar and all the recipes contain high levels of helpful nutrients to alleviate the symptoms of PMS.

First, a few words of advice. Premenstrual days are not, in general, a good time to be in the kitchen. During the few days in each month when women are most prone to accidents, it is unwise to put yourself in a situation where you are likely to smash your best china, burn yourself, slice off a finger, and so on.

Furthermore, remember that if anything goes wrong, as recipes sometimes do, it will cause you disappointment and frustration that is very much more intense than usual. So don't even think about making a soufflé, for example.

Successful eating premenstrually depends on getting the balance right between:

* Following sound nutritional principles designed to help minimise the troublesome symptoms.
* Using sensible strategies to make meal preparation as safe and hassle-free as possible.

The recipes that follow are specially selected to ensure that you spend as little time as possible in the kitchen during the most difficult days of the month, and that this time is well spent making meals that are nutritious, tasty and simple.

Some General Hints

* When cooking rice, pasta or potatoes, make an extra portion or two to keep in the fridge for later. If you're hit by late-night (or any other) munchies this will be a healthy, filling, snack that needs no preparation.

* When making meals during your 'good' days, remember to make extra batches of favourite family meals to freeze, so that you can reproduce them with a minimum of work on the 'bad' days.

* Plan ahead for difficult days. Time your supermarket mega-shop so that you are well stocked up with bread (pop a couple of extra wholemeal loaves in the freezer so you are sure not to run out) and a supply of foods for snacks that will fill you up without upsetting your blood sugar levels.

* If premenstrual bingeing is a problem, avoid temptation – don't keep stores of biscuits and sweets in the house, or at least not at danger times. This needn't mean depriving your sweet-toothed offspring; just buy them their sweets when they are going to eat them. Weaning them onto fresh fruit instead is, of course, a healthier alternative.

* On the subject of sweet things, although dried fruit is more nourishing than a highly processed sugary snack, it is also a concentrated source of sugars. So don't fool yourself! If you just switch from biscuits to shovelling handfuls of raisins into your mouth, you have not progressed much in terms of improving your diet.

* It may be worthwhile investing in a blender or liquidiser, as this will help you to make delicious and nutritious fresh fruit juices and soups in no time at all. When making soups, always make more than you need, and freeze it in individual portion sizes, so that you can easily heat some up whenever you feel like it.

Larder Essentials

Have a good supply of these on hand and you shouldn't have to resort to anything that upsets your blood sugar levels too much:

Rice cakes; wheat crackers

Breakfast cereal with no added sugar; oats

Potatoes; brown rice; pasta (preferably wholemeal)

Wholemeal bread; baked goods containing sodium-free baking powder (potassium bicarbonate); rye bread (if wheat is a problem food); soda bread or unleavened bread (if yeast is a problem food)

Soya flour; cracked wheat (bulgar wheat); buckwheat noodles; pot barley; lentils; chick peas

Fresh oily fish, such as mackerel, herring, sardines, salmon and trout; tinned tuna in soya oil or olive oil

Meat, preferably organic; free-range chicken; chicken liver

Skimmed or semi-skimmed milk

Free-range eggs

Low-sodium cheese

Unsalted butter; low-sodium peanut butter

Low-sodium mayonnaise

Unsalted nuts, such as almonds and hazelnuts; sunflower seeds (great to snack on)

Olive oil

Fresh or dried herbs: basil, chives, dill, fennel, garlic, mint, nutmeg, fresh onion, oregano, rosemary, sage, tarragon, thyme, turmeric

Tamari or soy sauce

Baked beans with no added sugar

Low-sodium mineral water

Fresh vegetables – including avocados, asparagus, spinach and other leafy vegetables

Fresh fruit – a wide selection including apples and banana, which make great snacks.

Meals and Snacks Away from Home

When hunger strikes at work, or out and about, it can be tempting to grab a chocolate bar or other unsuitable snack. Here are some of the better choices:

Banana or apple (but avoid over-sweet fruit)
Crispbreads
Rice cakes
Thin wheat crackers
Plain wheat biscuits
A small packet of unsalted nuts
Cereal bar containing oats and nuts
Flap-jack made from oats and honey.

Recipes

I have roughly classified these by the time of day you might choose to eat them, but there is no need to stick to this rigidly. So long as you avoid going for more than three hours or so without food, any of the following should be suitable for most times of day.

SUNNY BREAKFASTS
Super Seed Shake
This fast milk-shake is full of calcium and iron and the seeds contain healthy EFAs.

Serves 2

1 level tbsp sunflower seeds
1 level tbsp sesame seeds
300ml (½ pint) skimmed milk, soya milk or apple juice
1tsp crude blackstrap molasses
1 ripe banana, peeled

Finely grind the sunflower and sesame seeds in a coffee mill or similar. Blend the ground seeds, milk or apple juice, molasses and banana together.

Buckwheat Pancakes

These tasty pancakes are a rich source of B vitamins and magnesium. Try them with some real maple syrup and lemon juice, or roll them round a large spoonful of low-fat fromage frais. For a savoury filling, try stir-fried vegetable strips sprinkled with tamari sauce.

Serves 6/makes about 20 pancakes

100g (4oz) buckwheat flour
100g (4oz) brown rice flour
2 free-range eggs (size 3), lightly beaten
600ml (1 pint) soya milk
2tbsp sesame or olive oil for frying

Preheat the oven to 120°C (gas mark 2, 250°F).

Sift the flours together in a basin and make a well in the centre. Add the beaten egg and gradually beat in the soya to make a smooth batter. Leave the batter to stand for 30 minutes.

To cook the pancakes, stir the batter, then heat a little oil in a frying pan. Quickly pour in a tablespoon of batter to coat the base of the pan thinly. Cook the pancake until light brown underneath, then flip it over with a palette knife or fish slice and cook the other side. Slide the pancake onto a warmed heatproof dish, roll it up (with any filling) and place in the oven to keep warm. Continue making the remaining pancakes in the same way.

Hot Bulgar Breakfast

This delicious, nutritious hot cereal is a perfect winter-warmer and it is also rich in nutrients such as vitamins B6 and E, chromium and EFAs. Serve plain or with a little additional milk or soya milk.

Serves 4

> 1tbsp olive oil
> 150g (5oz) bulgar wheat (cracked wheat)
> 100g (4oz) sesame seeds
> 600ml (1 pint) water
> 100g (4oz) wheatgerm
> 25g (1oz) dried apricots, finely chopped
> 25g (1oz) raisins or currants
> 25g (1oz) chopped hazelnuts or almonds

Gently heat the oil in a large saucepan, add the bulgar wheat, sesame seeds and wheatgerm, and lightly sauté until slightly browned. Add the water and stir in the dried fruits. Cover and simmer for about 25 minutes, or until the bulgar is fluffy and the water has been absorbed. Add the nuts to taste and serve immediately.

Bircher Muesli

This nutritious recipe is based on the original invented by Dr Bircher-Benner for patients at his famous natural health clinic in Switzerland. To save time in the mornings, the oats may be soaked overnight, leaving only the fruit and hazelnuts to be added at breakfast.

Serves 2

> 4tbsp rolled oats
> 2tbsp low-fat, live yoghurt
> 6tbsp cold water
> 1/2tsp grated lemon rind
> 225g (8oz) freshly grated (unpeeled) apple, or 450g (1lb)
>   seasonal soft fruits
> 2tbsp chopped hazelnuts

Put the oats, yoghurt, water and lemon rind into a large bowl and stir until creamy. Leave in the fridge overnight if preferred. Add the fruit and serve sprinkled with the chopped hazelnuts.

More Breakfast Suggestions

*   Drink a glass of freshly squeezed fruit juice, or hot water and a slice of lemon, instead of tea or coffee in the morning
*   Try wholegrain cereal with semi-skimmed/skimmed milk and no added sugar, with sliced apple or banana
*   Spread two pieces of wholemeal toast with sunflower margarine and Marmite (unless you are prone to *Candida*) or peanut butter. To make your own nut butter, see **Light Lunches**.

ELEVENSES

*   Apple rolled in sesame seeds
*   Unsalted nuts and raisins
*   Banana
*   Rice cakes with Marmite or low-salt peanut butter
*   Thin slice of low-salt cheese on a wholewheat cracker
*   Slice of wholemeal bread with some humus, mushroom pâté or chicken liver pâté (see Light Lunches).

LIGHT LUNCHES

Tuna-stuffed Pitta Pocket

This tasty combination of tuna and onion makes a light meal and can be packed into a lunch box. Spring onion may be used in place of regular onions.

Serves 1

> *50g (2oz) tuna, packed in brine*
> *1tbsp onion, finely chopped*
> *2tbsp alfalfa sprouts*
> *2tsp low-sodium mayonnaise or low-fat fromage frais*
> *a dash of lemon juice and freshly ground black pepper to season*
> *1 wholemeal pitta bread*
> *2 lettuce leaves, shredded*

Mix together the tuna, onion, alfalfa sprouts and mayonnaise and add the seasoning. Slice the pitta bread in half and create two pockets. Line each pocket with shredded lettuce and stuff with the tuna fish mixture.

Warm Goat's Cheese Salad

Goat's cheese is more easily digested than cheese made from cow's milk, as its fat and protein molecules are much smaller. The sunflower seeds are rich in B vitamins and vitamin E as well as protein, and the dressing contains nutritious herbs.

Serves 4

> 175g (6oz) goat's cheese
> 1tbsp cold-pressed olive oil
> 16 mixed salad leaves
> 50g (2oz) sunflower seeds
> 2tbsp Fine French Dressing (see Delicious Dressings, at
>   the end of this chapter)

Preheat the oven to 180°C (gas mark 4, 350°F) or use the grill.

Slice the goat's cheese into four. Brush a baking tray with the olive oil and place the cheese slices on it. Heat in the oven or under a medium grill until lightly browned. Meanwhile, toss the salad leaves in the dressing and arrange on four small plates. Place one slice of goat's cheese in the centre. Sprinkle with sunflower seeds and serve immediately.

Vitamin Salad

This salad can be adapted to include any of your favourite raw vegetables. Vitamin salad is especially good served with Orange and Tamari Dressing (see Delicious Dressings, at the end of this Chapter). In order to maintain your energy levels, it is important to eat some complex carbohydrate with the salad, such as a baked potato or a wholemeal bread roll.

Serves 4–6

    50g (2oz) Brussels sprouts, grated
    50g (2oz) parsnip, peeled and grated
    50g (2oz) swede, peeled and grated
    50g (2oz) raw beetroot, grated
    50g (2oz) olives, finely diced
    50g (2oz) cabbage, shredded
    50g (2oz) celery, chopped
    1 small onion, peeled and finely chopped
    50g (2oz) watercress or mustard and cress
    salad dressing of your choice

Mix all the ingredients together in a large bowl and stir in your favourite dressing.

Tabbouleh

This Lebanese salad dish is light but filling and can be eaten on its own or with some fish or chicken.

    Serves 6
    175g (6oz) bulgar wheat
    1 medium-sized cucumber, diced
    4 spring onions, trimmed and finely chopped
    1–2tbsp freshly chopped basil
    1–2tbsp freshly chopped mint
    4tbsp freshly chopped parsley
    freshly squeezed juice of 1 lemon
    4tbsp cold-pressed olive oil or unrefined hazelnut oil
    For the garnish
    6 slivers red pepper or pimento
    6 chopped black olives

Rinse the bulgar wheat thoroughly before soaking it in cold water for at least an hour. Drain well.

Add the cucumber, spring onions and herbs to the lemon juice and oil and mix together well. Pour the mixture over the bulgar wheat and stir thoroughly. Serve garnished with slivers of red pepper or pimento and chopped black olives.

Salad Niçoise

I have omitted the anchovies from this traditional French recipe because of their high sodium content. The tuna and eggs are a valuable source of vitamin B6.

Serves 4

>1 crisp lettuce, washed and separated into leaves
>1 tin of tuna in soya or olive oil, drained (or fresh tuna)
>1tbsp fresh basil, chopped
>1tbsp fresh parsley, chopped
>175g (6oz) green beans, cooked
>½ cucumber, sliced
>500g (1lb) ripe tomatoes, sliced
>2tbsp (60ml) Fine French Dressing (see Delicious
>   Dressings, at the end of this chapter)
>4 free-range eggs, hard boiled

Line a bowl or plate with the lettuce leaves and flake the tuna over the centre. Then add half the chopped herbs, the green beans, sliced cucumber and tomato. Toss the ingredients with the dressing and garnish with quarters of hard boiled eggs and the remaining herbs.

Buckwheat Noodle Soup

A satisfying soup made with nourishing noodles and kombu seaweed (kelp).

Serves 2–3

>2.75l (5 pints) water, plus 350ml (12fl oz) water
>225g (8oz) buckwheat noodles
>8 spring onions, trimmed and finely chopped
>1tbsp olive oil
>750ml (1¼ pints) water
>3 inch piece of kombu seaweed
>3tbsp tamari sauce

Bring 2.75l (5 pints) water to the boil in a large saucepan. Add the buckwheat noodles and bring the water back to the boil, then add 12ml (4fl oz) cold water. Repeat the process twice. Take the saucepan off the heat, cover and leave for 10 minutes. Drain and rinse the noodles in cold water and set aside.

Heat the oil in a saucepan and sauté the spring onions for a few minutes. Add 750ml (1¼ pints) water and the seaweed, and bring to the boil. Cover and simmer for 15 minutes. Remove the seaweed and set on one side. Stir the tamari sauce into the soup and bring back to the boil. Meanwhile reheat the noodles by pouring boiling water over them. Drain and put the noodles into warmed bowls with the seaweed, and pour the soup over.

Barley and Vegetable Soup

A hearty, nourishing soup that satisfies the hungriest of stomachs. This recipe works particularly well with root vegetables, such as carrot, parsnip and swede.

Serves 4

> 3tbsp cold-pressed olive oil
> 2 onions, peeled and chopped
> 450g (1lb) any vegetable, chopped, diced or shredded
> 75g (3oz) pot barley
> ½tsp freshly grated root ginger
> 1.2l (2 pints) vegetable stock
> freshly ground black pepper

In a large saucepan, heat the oil and lightly sauté the onions and the vegetable of your choice. Stir in the pot barley, root ginger and stock and season with the pepper. Cover and simmer over a low heat for 2 hours, or until the barley is soft.

FILLINGS FOR SANDWICHES, BAKED POTATOES, ETC
Humus

This is a delicious filling and is very tasty on rye crackers and rice cakes.

Serves 2–4

> *50g (2oz) cooked chick peas*
> *juice of 1 lemon*
> *2 cloves garlic, peeled and crushed*
> *1tbsp cold-pressed olive oil*
> *1tbsp tahini*
> *50ml (2fl oz) water (optional)*
>
> For the garnish
> *1tbsp fresh parsley, chopped*
> *1tbsp pine kernels (nuts)*

If using a food processor, place all the ingredients in the container and blend until smooth. Alternatively, place all the ingredients into a large mixing bowl and pound with a potato masher, if necessary adding a little water to make the mixture smooth. Serve garnished with parsley and pine nuts.

Avocado and Alfalfa Sandwich Filling

A luxurious sandwich recipe which will fill you up with goodness. Avocado is a rich source of vitamin E and the alfalfa sprouts contain calcium and B vitamins.

Alfalfa sprouts are highly nutritious and they can be bought already sprouted from most supermarkets, or you can sprout them yourself at home. To do this, simply place a heaped tablespoon of alfalfa seeds in a clean jam jar or pot. Cover the top with a clean, disposable wiping cloth or piece of muslin and secure with an elastic band. Run some cold water into the covered jar, invert it and let the water drain away. Repeat this rinsing several times a day until the seeds have sprouted.

Note that all sprouting seeds achieve maximum sweetness just after they have sprouted. Once leaves start to form, the sugars are converted progressively into acids and cellulose.

Serves 1
> *1/2 avocado*
> *1/2 spring onion, finely chopped*
> *dash of lemon juice*

freshly ground black pepper
large handful alfalfa sprouts
2 slices of wholemeal bread

Mash the avocado with the spring onion, lemon juice and black pepper and spread on a slice of bread. Sprinkle with the alfalfa sprouts and top with the second slice of bread.

Tahini and Cucumber Sandwich Filling

This is an instant and tasty snack. Tahini spread is made from crushed sesame seeds. It is very high in calcium and is available from good supermarkets and health-food shops. Sesame seeds are high in fat.

Serves 1

¹/₂tbsp tahini spread
1tsp chopped parsley
6 cucumber slices
2 slices of wholemeal bread

Spread the tahini onto one of the slices of bread. Sprinkle on the chopped parsley and place the cucumber and second slice of bread on top. Serve with cherry tomatoes, radishes and spring onions.

Nut Butter

Nut butter and celery make an unusual and tasty filling for sandwiches and baked potatoes. But nut butter is far more versatile than just a spread – try dabbing a little over cooked carrots, or adding a tsp to a salad dressing for extra flavour. A more dilute form, usually made with ground almonds and water, is known as nut cream, and can be a nutritious (if fattening) substitute for milk. Nuts are a good source of vitamin E and healthy, polyunsaturated oil. Nuts are also rich in important minerals such as zinc and iron.

450g (1lb) mixture of almonds, brazil nuts, walnuts,
hazelnuts or peanuts
4tbsp apple juice

Roast the nuts in a medium oven for 10–15 minutes, stirring occasionally. Grind to a fine paste in a coffee mill or food processor with a sharp blade. Stir in just enough apple juice to make a thick purée. Store in screw-top jars. If the natural oil in the nuts separates, simply stir it back in. You can also make this recipe using seeds. For seeds such as sesame or sunflower, dry roast in a pan over a low heat until the seeds crush easily when rubbed. Then proceed as before. If any nut paste, particularly peanut, should become mouldy, dispose of immediately.

Peanut Butter Specials

Peanut butter is a staple sandwich spread. Rich in vitamin E, it works well with many other ingredients to create extra special sandwich fillings. Try these combinations:

* Smooth peanut butter and cucumber
* Smooth peanut butter and sliced apple
* Crunchy peanut butter with alfalfa sprouts and celery
* Crunchy peanut butter with cottage cheese and pineapple.

Mushroom Pâté

This is very useful as a sandwich filling, or spread on rice cakes as a starter or snack. I find that the larger varieties of mushrooms have more flavour.

Serves 4–6

>   1tbsp cold-pressed olive oil
>   225g (8oz) mushrooms, roughly chopped
>   1 clove garlic, peeled and crushed
>   2tbsp white wine
>   50g (2oz) almonds or hazelnuts
>   2tbsp very low-fat fromage frais
>   For the garnish
>   slivers of red and yellow sweet peppers

Heat the oil in a large frying pan and briefly fry the mushrooms and garlic before adding the white wine. Simmer until the mushrooms are cooked and the liquid has been absorbed. Place the mixture in a food processor with the almonds or hazelnuts and blend into a coarse paste. Fold in the fromage frais and chill before serving, garnished with the peppers.

Low-fat Chicken Liver Pâté

Chicken liver is a rich source of iron, vitamin B6 and zinc – all of which may help to alleviate the symptoms of PMS. This low-fat recipe is delicious and can be used as a starter or as a sandwich filling.

Serves 4

> 1tbsp olive oil
> 1 onion, chopped
> 1 clove garlic, crushed
> 200g (7oz) chicken livers
> ½ glass of red wine or vegetable stock
> salt and pepper to season
> 2tbsp wholegrain mustard

Sauté the onion and garlic in olive oil, add the chicken livers. Cook until browned before adding the red wine or vegetable stock. Season with salt, pepper and wholegrain mustard. Cook for 10–15 minutes. Chop finely or purée in a food processor, cool and serve with toast, crackers or a salad of carrot and celery.

AFTERNOON FILLERS

Nice Rice Pudding

This wonderfully warming pudding should give you a boost in the afternoon and it gets most of its sweetness from the rice. It is important to use precooked rice.

Serves 4

    100g (4oz) cooked sweet brown rice
    ½tbsp clear honey or ½tbsp dried fruit, such as sultanas,
       chopped apricots or dates
    600ml (1 pint) soya milk
    pinch of freshly grated nutmeg

Preheat the oven to 150°C (gas mark 2, 300°F).

    Place the precooked rice in a lightly oiled ovenproof dish. Stir the honey or the dried fruit into the milk and pour over the rice. Sprinkle on the fresh nutmeg. Bake for approximately two hours.

Courgette and Carrot Cake

This rich, dark cake tastes so delicious you won't believe it's so good for you! Less sweet than conventional recipes, it is enriched with vitamin E and iron. Butter is replaced with healthier monounsaturated oil which also makes the mixture fabulously moist. I add coarsely chopped walnut pieces for extra crunch. It shouldn't send your blood glucose levels soaring.

    Makes two 18cm (7 inch) cakes

    2 free-range eggs, size 3
    2tbsp crude blackstrap molasses
    2tbsp clear honey
    150ml (¼ pint) plus 1tbsp walnut, hazelnut or olive oil
    175g (6oz) buckwheat flour
    1tsp bicarbonate of soda
    50g (2oz) natural wheatgerm
    100g (4oz) carrots, scrubbed and grated
    100g (4oz) courgettes, washed and grated
    50g (2oz) chopped walnuts
    4tbsp orange juice

Preheat the oven to 180°C (gas mark 4, 350°F).

    Lightly oil two sponge sandwich tins with 1tbsp of oil. In a large mixing bowl, beat the eggs together before adding the molasses and honey. Stir vigorously before pouring in 150ml (¼ pint) of oil. Fold in the buckwheat flour, bicarbonate of soda and wheatgerm, followed by the remaining ingredients. Pour into the baking tins and bake for 35–40 minutes, or until a metal skewer comes out clean. Allow to cool before turning out and slicing into wedges. Store in a tightly sealed container in a cool place.

Wheat-free Fruit and Nut Loaf

This delicious loaf is just right for those who find that wheat causes bloating and other symptoms of PMS.

> 100g (4oz) low-sodium butter/margarine
> 100g (4oz) unrefined sugar (reduced to superfine texture in a food processor)
> 2 free-range eggs
> 200g (5½oz) wheat-free self-raising flour
> 75g (3oz) mixed raisins and sultanas
> 75g (3oz) walnuts, sliced

Preheat the oven to 190°C (gas mark 4, 375°F).

Gently mix together the butter and sugar until light and fluffy. Add the eggs and gradually fold in the flour. Then add the fruit and nuts and stir. Pour the mixture into a 500g (1lb) cake tin and bake in the oven for 20–25 minutes.

Spiced Bananas

This recipe works well with pears too. Another way to make this dish is to bake the fruit in a preheated oven at 180°C (gas mark 4, 350°F) for 15 minutes to soften it, before pouring on the sauce and serving. Bake the bananas in their skins and they'll keep their colour better.

Serves 4

> 4 large ripe bananas
> 50g (2oz) butter or soya margarine
> 1tbsp clear honey
> 2tsp allspice

Peel and slice the bananas and place in four individual serving bowls. In a small saucepan, quickly melt the butter or soya margarine, and stir in the honey and allspice. Pour over the bananas and serve immediately.

More Afternoon Snacks
* Banana or apple
* Wholemeal toast with peanut butter, Marmite or honey
* Rice cakes with peanut butter
* Low-sodium cheese and wholemeal crackers
* Unsalted nuts and raisins

DINNERS
Home-made Herb Sausages
These brilliant bangers can be made with either lamb or pork. They are lower in fat than the shop varieties and do not contain any additives. The pork sausages must be cooked all the way through, but the lamb sausages may be left slightly pink inside. Meat and eggs are both good sources of vitamin B6, which can help in the treatment of PMS.

Makes 8–10 sausages
olive oil, for frying (optional)
450g (1lb)lean lamb or pork, diced or minced
1 small onion, peeled and roughly chopped
1tsp French mustard
1 free-range egg, size 3
25g (1oz) buckwheat flour or barley flour for coating
For the lamb sausages
4 large sprigs of fresh mint or basil, roughly chopped
For the pork sausages
4 large sprigs of fresh sage, roughly chopped

Mix all the ingredients together in a food processor until the mixture resembles sausage meat (this may take a few minutes). Divide the mixture into eight portions and, with floured hands, roll each into a sausage shape. The bangers can either be shallow fried in a little olive oil or cooked under a medium grill.

Majestic Mince

This filling recipe replaces the saturated fat content of the minced meat with healthier vegetable oils. Serve with baked potatoes, brown rice or wholewheat pasta shells.

Serves 3–4

> 225g (8oz) lean minced beef or lamb (preferably
>   organically reared)
> 3tbsp olive oil or sunflower oil
> ¼ small cabbage, chopped
> 4 carrots, thinly sliced
> 2 leeks, thinly sliced
> 1tsp fresh oregano, chopped
> 1tsp fresh rosemary, chopped
> 450g (1lb) tomatoes, chopped, or 400g (14oz) tin chopped
>   tomatoes
> freshly ground black pepper

Put the mince in a microwave oven, or in a heavy-based saucepan on top of the stove, and heat until cooked. Pour all the meat juices and fat into a basin, and set on one side to cool. Skim off the fat and pour only the juices back into the meat.

Gently heat the olive or sunflower oil in a saucepan and add the vegetables. Cover and simmer for 5 minutes or until the vegetables are soft. Add the mince, herbs, tomatoes, and pepper to season. Simmer for a further 5 minutes to allow the full flavour to develop.

Fast Fish Risotto

This is a good way to use precooked rice, and the frozen peas are an excellent source of fibre and protein. Tinned fish, such as tuna or salmon, may be substituted for the fresh oily fish.

Serves 2

100g (4oz) fresh oily fish (eg mackerel or herring)
1tbsp olive oil
1 onion, peeled and finely chopped
6 heaped tbsp cooked brown rice
150g (5oz) frozen peas
1tbsp fresh basil or parsley, chopped

Cook the fresh fish under a hot grill for about 5 minutes, turning once. Allow to cool slightly, then flake into large pieces.

Heat the oil in a large frying pan and lightly fry the onion. Add the fresh or tinned fish, rice and peas. Stir continuously to prevent the mixture sticking to the sides of the pan, while heating through for about 3 minutes. Garnish with the chopped basil or parsley before serving.

Really Easy Roast Chicken

Chicken is a good source of vitamin B6, zinc and protein. This recipe is very simple and it tastes great with the apricot stuffing. Try to use free-range chicken, if available, as it is healthier and tastier too.

Serves 4-6

1 fresh free-range chicken (about 1.75kg/4lb)
1tbsp cold-pressed olive oil
2tbsp fresh mixed herbs, chopped, or 1tbsp dried mixed herbs
freshly ground black pepper
Apricot Stuffing (see opposite)

Preheat the oven to 200°C (gas mark 5, 400°F).

Place the chicken in a roasting tray. Brush with the olive oil and sprinkle with the herbs and pepper. Cover with foil and roast in the oven for 20 minutes per 1lb plus 20–30 minutes uncovered. Baste the chicken occasionally. To test if it's cooked, insert a skewer into the thickest part of the thigh. The juices should run clear. Allow the chicken to stand in a warm place for 10 minutes before carving.

Apricot Stuffing
To stuff one 1.75kg (4lb) chicken

175g (6oz) dried apricots, chopped
175g (6oz) fresh, wholewheat breadcrumbs
1/2tsp lemon juice
4tbsp cold-pressed olive oil
freshly ground black pepper

Soak the apricots in cold water for about 30 minutes, or until plump and soft. Stir in the breadcrumbs. Add the lemon juice, olive oil and pepper to season. Work some of the stuffing firmly over the breast and secure the neckflap to keep the stuffing in place. Spoon the remaining stuffing inside the cavity of the chicken.

Seafood Spears

Choose fish with a firm flesh, such as cod, tuna or salmon, so that it will thread easily onto skewers. Serve on a bed of mixed brown and wild rices.

Serves 4

For the marinade
4tbsp unrefined sunflower or safflower oil
juice of 1 lemon
1tbsp tamari sauce
1tbsp fresh parsley, chopped
freshly ground black pepper

For the spears
750g (1¹/2lb) fresh or frozen fish
8 scallops or large prawns
8 shallots, peeled, or 2 large onions, peeled and quartered
¹/2 red and ¹/2 green sweet pepper, deseeded and diced
*   roughly*
2 courgettes, thickly sliced

For the garnish
1tbsp fresh parsley, chopped

Combine the ingredients for the marinade. Blanch the shallots or onions for 1 minute in boiling water.

Cut the fish into chunks and steep in the marinade for half an hour. Thread, together with the scallops or prawns, shallots or onions, peppers and courgettes, onto wooden or metal skewers. Brush with the marinade, place under a medium grill and cook for about 5 minutes (depending upon the fish). Turn the kebabs twice, brushing them with marinade as they cook. Garnish with chopped parsley before serving.

Prawn Kebabs with Herb Marinade

These tasty kebabs can be served with brown rice or Tabouleh (see Light Lunches)

> **Serves 2**
> *For the kebabs*
>> *12 king-sized prawns*
>> *8 button mushrooms*
>> *1 medium courgette, sliced*
> *For the herb marinade*
>> *4tbsp olive or sunflower oil*
>> *1 clove garlic, peeled and crushed*
>> *juice of 1 lemon*
>> *1 sprig each of basil, parsley and tarragon, finely chopped*

Thread the prawns, button mushrooms and sliced courgettes onto wooden or metal skewers and place in a shallow dish. Mix the marinade ingredients together and pour over the kebabs. Cover and leave to marinate for 30 minutes. Place under a medium grill for about 5 minutes, basting and turning the kebabs as they cook.

Halibut with Watercress Sauce

Halibut is ideal for baking because it has a firm texture and doesn't fall apart as you transfer it to a plate. A whole halibut can weigh up to 300lb, which means that the steaks are large enough to satisfy the heartiest appetites.

Serves 4

1 small onion, finely chopped
150ml (¼ pint) dry white wine
1kg (approx 2lb) halibut steaks
1tbsp olive oil
100g (4oz) watercress, chopped
1tsp smooth mustard
freshly ground black pepper

Preheat the oven to 230°C (gas mark 6, 450°F)

Place the onions and white wine in a casserole dish or stainless steel baking kettle (with a lid). Lay the halibut steaks on top and drizzle with olive oil. Cover and bake in the oven for 15–20 minutes until almost cooked through. Move the fish to a hot serving dish and cover with a piece of foil to keep warm. Transfer the cooking juices to a small saucepan, add the chopped watercress and boil for about 1 minute. Use a hand-held blender (or transfer to a food processor) to purée the sauce. Add the mustard and pepper to taste and pour over the halibut just before serving.

Stuffed Red Peppers

A no-fuss supper dish that looks impressive but takes no time to put together. It is another great way of using up left-over rice. Serve with spring greens or spinach.

Serves 4

1 medium onion, finely chopped
50ml (2fl oz) olive oil
100g (4oz) mushrooms, finely chopped
1 medium sized carrot, finely chopped
2 mugs of cooked brown rice
400g (14oz) tin of chopped tomatoes
¼tsp dried mixed herbs
freshly ground black pepper

> *4 large red sweet peppers*
> *100g (4oz) grated cheddar cheese*
> *1tbsp basil, chopped*

Preheat the oven to 190°C (gas mark 4, 375°F).

In a large pan, lightly fry the onion in the olive oil, then add the mushrooms and carrot and stir well. Add the chopped tomatoes, mixed herbs and black pepper. Bring to the boil and simmer until the liquid reduces. Meanwhile prepare the peppers by removing their stalks (push the stalks down into the pepper, twist and remove). Rinse the seeds out from inside each one. Add the rice to the tomato sauce and mix well. Balance the peppers alongside each other in a casserole dish or baking tin and stuff with the rice mixture. Sprinkle the grated cheese over the tops of each pepper and bake in the oven for 15–20 minutes. Serve garnished with the chopped basil.

BEDTIME SNACKS

Women often experience insomnia before their period arrives, and eating some form of complex carbohydrate before going to bed can help prevent this. Although it is not easy to fall asleep on an empty stomach, it is not a good idea to sleep on a full one either. It is important to let your body digest a large meal before going to bed. It is also not a good idea to eat very spicy or acidic foods before going to bed, as your stomach may have problems digesting these and this could keep you awake. Cheese is another food to avoid at bedtime as it is difficult to digest – remember the old wives' tale about cheese causing nightmares! Here are some ideas for bedtime snacks which should soon send you off to sleep:

* Rice cakes spread with peanut butter or Marmite
* Slice of wholemeal bread and sunflower spread
* Piece of toast and honey
* Bowl of sliced banana in low-fat live yoghurt
* Small bowl of cereal with skimmed milk.

DELICIOUS DRESSINGS

Fine French Dressing

Stored sealed in the fridge, this dressing will keep for up to a week.

Makes 300ml (¼ pint)

> 1–2 large cloves garlic, peeled and crushed
> ¼tsp freshly grated root ginger
> 120ml (4fl oz) lemon juice
> ½tsp mustard
> 175ml (6fl oz) unrefined sunflower or safflower oil
> freshly ground black pepper

Put all the ingredients together in a screw-top jar, replace the lid and shake vigorously to mix well.

Cucumber Dressing

A delicious, refreshing dressing that works well on baked potatoes and sliced avocados.

Serves 2-4

> 1tbsp cider vinegar
> 150g (5oz) cucumber
> 1 sprig of dill
> ½tsp dried dill seeds
> 150g (5oz) natural low-fat, live yoghurt

Blend all the ingredients together in a food processor until the dressing is smooth and creamy.

Yoghurt and Chive Dressing

Serves 2–4

> 2tbsp chopped chives
> 1 clove garlic, peeled and crushed
> 1tbsp lemon juice
> 1tsp Dijon mustard
> 1tbsp cold-pressed olive oil
> 150ml (¼ pint) natural low-fat, live yoghurt
> freshly ground black pepper

In a large bowl, mix all the ingredients together, adding pepper
to season, and stir vigorously. Alternatively, place the ingredients in a large, screw-top jar, replace the lid and shake well.

Orange and Tamari Dressing

This is very good with green-leaf vegetables such as spinach, or
salad leaves. It is also a useful dressing for those who dislike
vinegar.

Serves 2-4

> *1 clove garlic, peeled and crushed*
> *1tsp finely chopped fresh root ginger*
> *3tbsp olive oil*
> *150ml (¼ pint) freshly squeezed orange juice*
> *1tsp grated orange peel*
> *2tbsp tamari sauce*

In a large bowl, mix all the ingredients together and stir well
before using. Alternatively, place the ingredients in a large,
screw-top jar, replace the lid and shake well.

Appendix 1

Menstrual Chart

NAME								YEAR				

	JAN	FEB	MAR	APR	MAY	JUNE	JULY	AUG	SEP	OCT	NOV	DEC
1												
2												
3												
4												
5												
6												
7												
8												
9												
10												
11												
12												
13												
14												
15												
16												
17												
18												
19												
20												
21												
22												
23												
24												
25												
26												
27												
28												
29												
30												
31												

SUGGESTED KEY TO SYMBOLS:
M (or red line) = Menstruation   P = Panic attack
B = Breast tenderness   A = Asthma attack
W = Fluid retention   D = Depression
I = Irritability   H = Headache

Appendix 2
PMS Treatment Options

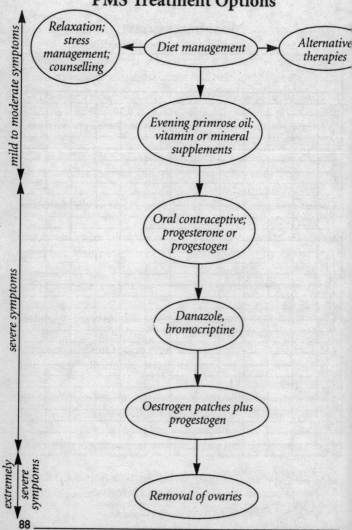

mild to moderate symptoms

severe symptoms

extremely severe symptoms

Relaxation; stress management; counselling

Diet management

Alternative therapies

Evening primrose oil; vitamin or mineral supplements

Oral contraceptive; progesterone or progestogen

Danazole, bromocriptine

Oestrogen patches plus progestogen

Removal of ovaries

Glossary

Adrenal glands – a pair of glands; one sits on top of each kidney. They secrete the hormone **adrenaline.**

Adrenaline – hormone secreted by the **adrenal glands** in response to danger or low blood sugar, sometimes called the 'fright or flight' hormone.

Antioxidant – nutrient, such as a vitamin, which protects against oxidation – a process which can have harmful consequences in the body.

Benign – harmless; non-malignant.

Bromocriptine – a drug which blocks the action of the hormone **prolactin**.

Caffeine – a stimulant found in coffee and, in smaller amounts, in tea, chocolate and cola drinks.

Candida albicans – a yeast which normally exists harmlessly in the body but which can occasionally overgrow and cause the condition thrush.

Cervix – the aperture at the base of the **uterus**, where it opens into the vagina.

Chromium – an important trace mineral, involved in control of blood sugar levels.

Cis-linoleic acid – an essential fatty acid, found in vegetable oils, which is the raw material eventually made into **prostaglandin E1**.

Corpus luteum – the empty follicle left on the surface of the ovary after an egg has been released, which goes on to secrete the hormone **progesterone**.

Cyclogest – a brand of **progesterone** preparation in the form of a pessary.

Danazole – a brand drug which blocks the action of the female sex hormones and which can, in high enough doses, suppress **ovulation**.

Diuretic – a drug which stimulates the passing of water.

Duphaston – a brand of **progestogen** (artificial **progesterone**) preparation.

Enzyme – a substance produced by the body that regulates biochemical reactions.

Essential fatty acid (EFA) – those constituents of fat which are needed for the synthesis of chemicals that have important functions in the body, and which have to be supplied by the diet. Some EFAs are converted by the body into hormones and hormone-like substances called **prostaglandins**.

Fallopian tube – part of the female reproductive system. The **uterus** has a pair of fallopian tubes attached to it, each of which ends at an ovary. They carry eggs from the ovaries to the uterus.

Follicle stimulating hormone (FSH) – a hormone secreted by the **pituitary gland**. It instructs the ovary to produce a ripened egg, and to secrete the sex hormone **oestrogen**.

Gamma-linolenic acid (GLA) – a fatty acid which is produced in the body as part of the process of making **prostaglandin E1**. It is also found in evening primrose oil.

Gestone – a brand of **progesterone** preparation that is administered by injection.

Glucagon – a hormone secreted in response to a fall in blood sugar levels, that stimulates a rise by releasing glucose from storage.

Glycogen – a form of carbohydrate used by the liver to store glucose.

Hypoglycaemia – a deficiency of glucose in the bloodstream which causes muscular weakness, mental confusion and sweating. It is commonly caused by not eating enough carbohydrates.

Insulin – a hormone secreted in response to a rise in blood sugar levels, that stimulates a fall by removing glucose from the blood and into storage.

Luteal phase – the second half of the menstrual cycle, during which **progesterone** is secreted by the **corpus luteum**. This is when PMS occurs.

Luteinising hormone (LH) – a hormone secreted by the **pituitary gland**, which stimulates the **corpus luteum** on the ovary to produce the sex hormone **progesterone**.

Mastalgia – severe breast pain.

Mefenamic acid – a painkiller, sometimes known under the brand name Ponstan.

Menopause – the end of a woman's reproductive years, marked by irregular periods and, frequently, hormonal imbalance resulting in physical and psychological symptoms.

Nystatin – brand name for an antifungal drug.

Oestrogen – a steroid hormone which controls female sexual development.

Ovulation – the release of a ripe egg from an ovary, which takes place every month about half-way through the menstrual cycle.

Peripheral neuropathy – a disease of the nervous system which can result from continued overdose of vitamin B6 (**pyridoxine**).

Pituitary gland – a small gland in the brain which secretes hormones. Among them are **prolactin**, which stimulates the breasts to produce milk for the newborn baby; and the hormones that control the secretion of the sex hormones by the ovaries.

Placebo – a dummy drug which will have no physical effect on patients. It is given to some patients in clinical trials so that the results of their treatment can be contrasted with the results of the patients taking the active drug.

Polyunsaturated fat – a group of fatty acids that includes the EFAs. 'Polyunsaturated' refers to a structural feature of the fat molecule.

Ponstan – brand name for a preparation of the painkiller mefenamic acid.

Primolut N – brand of **progestogen** (synthetic **progesterone**) preparation.

Progesterone – a steroid hormone which is responsible for preparing the inner lining of the womb for pregnancy.

Progestogen – synthetic **progesterone**.

Prolactin – a hormone secreted by the **pituitary gland** which stimulates the breasts to produce milk for a newborn baby. During the normal menstrual cycle it can cause breast pain and bloating.

Prostaglandin E1 – a hormone-like chemical which is needed in the regulation of a woman's normal hormone balance.

Pyridoxine – another name for vitamin B6.

Selenium – an essential trace mineral.

Synergy – a situation in which one element has its effect enhanced while in the presence of another – the two are said to work in *synergy*; alternatively one is said to have a *synergistic* effect upon the other.

Uterus – the womb.

Useful Addresses

Institute for Complementary Medicine
PO Box 194
London SE16 1QZ
Tel: 0171-237 5165

National Association for Premenstrual Syndrome (NAPS)
PO Box 72
Sevenoaks
Kent TN13 1XQ
Information line: 01732 741709

PMS Help
PO Box 160, St Albans
Herts AL1 4UQ

Premenstrual Society (Premsoc)
PO Box 429, Addlestone
Surrey KT15 1DZ

Women's Health Information Centre
52 Featherstone Street
London EC1
Tel: 0171-251 6580

The Women's Nutritional Advisory Service
PO Box 268, Lewes
East Sussex BN7 2QN
Tel: 01273 487366

For more information about Evening Primrose Oil call the
Evening Primrose Office on 0171-720 8596.

Index